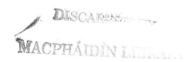

NUCLEAR MEDICINE FOR TECHNICIANS

NUCLEAR MEDICINE FOR TECHNICIANS

by ROBERT C. LANGE, PH.D.

Assistant Professor of Radiology
Yale University School of Medicine
Technical Director, Section of Nuclear Medicine
Yale-New Haven Hospital
New Haven, Connecticut

YEAR BOOK MEDICAL PUBLISHERS, INC.
35 East Wacker Drive · Chicago

Library of Congress Catalog Card Number: 72-95732
International Standard Book Number: 0-8151-5643-X

For Mary Anne, Lou and Chris

PREFACE

DURING THE PAST FEW YEARS, the specialty of nuclear medicine has taken a number of important steps in establishing its place as a diagnostic service to medicine. Among these steps has been the establishment of a number of schools designed to train nuclear medicine technicians and technologists. This book was written with these students in mind, but also with the hope that it would be useful for those technicians whose training in nuclear medicine was limited to on-the-job training. Heavy emphasis is placed on the physical sciences related to nuclear medicine, which is basic to the understanding of the processes by which diagnostic information is obtained in nuclear medicine.

I am indebted to many colleagues in the Section of Nuclear Medicine of the Yale University School of Medicine for support and assistance in preparing the manuscript, in particular Drs. Richard P. Spencer and Gerald S. Freedman. The assistance of Mrs. Agnes Farrar, Miss Grace Han, Mr. Bruce Kerrick, and Miss Gail Massella, technicians in the Section, is gratefully acknowledged. I am also indebted to Mrs. Greer Desjardin and Mrs. Carol Piscitelli for their unending patience and hard work in typing the manuscript. The illustrations were prepared by Mrs. Virginia Simon and her assistants, and their help was invaluable. Finally, I would like to express my appreciation to my wife Mary Anne and to my children for their patience and encouragement during the preparation of the manuscript.

Robert C. Lange

New Haven, Connecticut
May, 1972

Contents

CHAPTER 1

A Brief History of Nuclear Medicine

NUCLEAR MEDICINE CAN TRACE its development to the last decade of the nineteenth century, when Bequerel discovered the phenomenon of radioactivity. The years 1890 to 1900 were great years for experimental physics, for a number of new phenomena were observed for the first time. The importance of the discoveries and developments can be fairly judged by the fact that the Nobel Prizes, which were first awarded in 1901, were received predominantly by those scientists whose work had been completed before the turn of the century.

The x-ray (with "x" representing the unknown) had been discovered in 1895 by Wilhelm Röntgen (Nobel Prize for physics, 1901). Although the name x-ray has become well-established in English-speaking countries, the radiation is called Röntgen ray in most parts of the world. In fact, x-rays were found to have the characteristics of electromagnetic radiation (see Chap. 3) shortly after their discovery.

Bequerel's startling discovery of the ability of various uranium salts to fog photographic plates occurred in 1896, and within three years Pierre and Marie Curie had discovered two new elements (polonium and radium) solely by virtue of their radioactivity. These three scientists shared the Nobel Prize for physics in 1903. The term "radioactivity" was, in fact, coined by Marie Curie. The physical properties of one type of radiation (gamma rays) emitted by radioactive materials were soon found to be essentially identical with those of x-rays; that is, both gamma and x-rays are electromagnetic radiations with very short wavelengths.

Beginning in 1899, the British scientist Ernest Rutherford (Nobel Prize in chemistry, 1908) conducted a long series of experiments aimed at the identification of the radiations emitted by radioactive materials. Eventually the radiations (named alpha, beta and gamma, the first three letters of the Greek alphabet) were characterized as follows: alpha rays are helium nuclei, beta rays are electrons and gamma rays are short-wavelength electromagnetic radiation, as indicated above.

Until 1933, scientists with an interest in radioactive materials discovered a large number of naturally occurring radioactive elements. Most of these were heavy metals such as radium and polonium, and al-

1

though the radioactivity was put to a few practical uses—notably the use of radium implants in cancer therapy—for the most part the materials were laboratory curiosities. This is not to say that the work was fruitless; the discoveries of these 35 years had an enormous impact on theoretic ideas concerning the constitution of atoms and nuclei. The year 1933 was momentous because of the discovery of artificial radioactivity. Irène Curie (Marie's daughter) and Frédéric Joliot produced radioactive phosphorus by bombarding aluminum with alpha particles from an isotope of polonium.

With the development of the cyclotron by E. O. Lawrence (starting in 1931) and the discovery of the neutron by James Chadwick in 1934, it became possible to produce large numbers of artificial radioactive isotopes and to make them in fair quantity. However, it was not until the 1940s with the advent of nuclear reactors, a source of large numbers of neutrons, that it became practical to consider the possibility of producing large amounts of radioactive materials.

Nuclear medicine* probably originated with an investigation of the uptake of iodine 128 in the thyroid of the rabbit, performed in 1938 by a group headed by Robley D. Evans at the Massachusetts General Hospital and the Massachusetts Institute of Technology. For many years, the thyroid gland and thyroid carcinoma were the main concerns of nuclear medicine. The interest and usefulness of radioactive iodine have remained large in the practice of nuclear medicine, as witnessed by the number of diagnostic studies performed with this radioactive element even into the 1970s.

There are approximately 1,500 radioactive isotopes known today to physical scientists, but less than 20 have found any use in nuclear medicine. There are three properties of radioisotopes that are of prime importance in nuclear medicine. First is the physical half life, which is the time required for one half of the radioisotope to disappear by radioactive decay. In nuclear medicine, most studies are performed with short-lived (half life of a few days or less) materials, although radioisotopes with longer half lives are acceptable if they are not accumulated in the body. The desirability of short half lives is related to the radiation dose delivered to the patient, which, in the best of worlds, should be kept at a minimum.

The second important property of a medical radioisotope is the type of radiation emitted by the isotope. In order to localize an isotope within a patient's body or to measure the amount of radioactivity in a

---

* Nuclear medicine is one of the few things of the "atomic age" that is correctly named, since most of the phenomena—atom bombs, atomic reactors; *etc.*—are really associated with the *nucleus* of the atom.

biologic sample, the radiation must be detected outside the patient or sample. In general, this requirement means that the radioisotope must emit gamma rays, which can pass through the body or sample in a manner similar to x-rays. In nuclear medicine, the patient is the source of radiation, and special detectors are used to determine the distribution and amount of radioactive material in the body.

The third important characteristic of an isotope which is to be used in nuclear medicine is its interaction with the body. It should be noted that radioactive isotopes behave just like stable elements in the body, and that extremely small amounts of radioactive materials are administered. Thus, radioactive iodine is concentrated in the thyroid gland just as iodine is, although only about a billionth of a gram of radioactive iodine is administered to the patient. Sometimes it is necessary to incorporate the radioisotope into a chemical compound or a mixture which is handled only by a particular organ or cell type in the body, as in the case of liver scanning with colloidal particles tagged with a radioactive isotope.

For dynamic studies, which involve the flow of a radioisotope through or into an organ, the chemistry is not so important in the early phase of the examination, but must not be neglected, since the ultimate fate of the radioactive material in the body is of utmost importance in the radiation dose delivered to the patient.

The remaining chapters of this book are designed to provide the physical, chemical and medical information required by a nuclear medicine technologist in the performance of diagnostic examinations on patients and biologic samples. The first part deals primarily with the physics and chemistry of nuclear medicine, and the second part concentrates on clinical studies with radioisotopes.

SUGGESTED READING

Brucer, M.: *Thyroid Radioiodine Clinical Testing* (St. Louis: Mallinkrodt Chemical Works, 1969).

Curie, E.: *Marie Curie* (Translated by Vincent Sheean) Garden City, New York: Doubleday & Company, Inc., 1937).

Friedlander, G., Kennedy, J. W., and Miller, J. M.: *Nuclear and Radiochemistry* (2d ed.; New York: John Wiley and Sons, Inc., 1964), Chap. 1.

Jauncy, G. E. M.: The early years of radioactivity, Am. J. Physics, 14:226, 1946.

CHAPTER 2

Atomic and Nuclear Physics

The Atom and the Nucleus

Since the physical basis of nuclear medicine is the radiation resulting from the disintegration of unstable nuclei, understanding of the nucleus and the atom is of fundamental importance in the study of the technology of nuclear medicine. This chapter aims to provide the reader with sufficient details of atomic and nuclear structure so that the actual disintegration of nuclei (discussed in Chap. 5) can be understood.

Elements and the Nuclear Atom

The universe, so far as can be seen with the largest telescope, is made up of approximately 80 stable elements. That is, astronomers have been able to recognize familiar elements in the spectra of even the most distant stars. There have been no surprises in the materials (in the form of new elements) recently returned from the moon.

All elements have atoms. Atoms are the smallest subdivision of matter that can still be recognized as a particular element. Atoms themselves can be broken down into smaller, subatomic particles. There are three subatomic particles of interest. The *electrons* each carry one negative electric charge and are extremely small; electrons weigh 9.1×10^{-28} grams each. *Protons* carry one positive electric charge each, are much heavier (about 1,800 times) than electrons. Each proton weighs 1.7×10^{-24} grams. *Neutrons*, as the name implies, are electrically neutral. Neutrons weigh about the same as protons, but are slightly heavier.

The three subatomic particles are distributed in atoms in a particular way. Although no one has ever seen an atom, models have been developed which meet the pragmatic requirement of usefulness in explaining observed phenomena and in predicting the outcome of future experiments. Perhaps the best-known atomic model is that proposed by Nils Bohr in 1913. In the Bohr model, the atom is conceived as having most of its mass (weight) in an extremely small central region called the nucleus. The nucleus is where the protons and neutrons are. The electrons in the Bohr model are relegated to circular motion in orbits around the nucleus. The Bohr model of the sodium atom is shown in Figure 2-1.

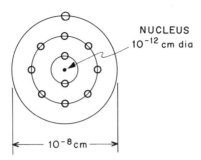

NUCLEUS
10^{-12} cm dia

$\longleftarrow 10^{-8}$ cm $\longrightarrow$

Fig. 2-1.— Bohr model of the sodium atom. The diameter of the atom is about one Angström (10^{-8} cm.), whereas the diameter of the nucleus is approximately 10^{-12} cm.

Later discussion will show that the Bohr model is not the best representation of the atomic structure, but it does serve as a good starting point in that it locates the heavy nucleus at the center of the atom and places the electrons outside.

The subatomic particles are of primary importance in establishing the identification of an element. Each element is identified by the number of protons in the nucleus; and since all atoms are electrically neutral, each element must have the same number of electrons as protons. For example, the neutral hydrogen atom has one proton in its nucleus, and one electron in its electron orbit. All uranium nuclei have 92 protons. Conversely, all atoms with 43 protons are technetium atoms. Elements are known for all proton numbers (often called Z, the atomic number) from 0 to 104. Elements with Z = 1 (hydrogen) to 42 (molybdenum), Z = 44 (ruthenium) to 60 (neodymium), and Z = 62 (samarium) to 83 (bismuth) have stable isotopes. Elements with Z = 0 (the neutron), 43 (technetium), 61 (promethium) and 84 (polonium) to 105 (as yet unnamed) are all unstable (radioactive).

Atomic Structure and Chemistry

For the most part, the chemical behavior of the various elements is governed by the number of electrons in the orbits, or shells, outside the nucleus. The arrangement of the electrons in the shells is of paramount importance, and is the basis of the periodic chart of the elements (see Fig. 2-2).

As mentioned earlier, the atoms of the elements are electrically neutral; the number of protons is equal to the number of electrons. Thus, hydrogen, which has one proton in the nucleus, has one electron in orbit around the nucleus; helium has two electrons, lithium three, and so on,

H																	He
Li	Be	B											C	N	O	F	Ne
Na	Mg	Al											Si	P	S	Cl	Ar
K	Ca	Sc	Ti	V	Cr	Mn	Fe	Co	Ni	Cu	Zn	Ga	Ge	As	Se	Br	Kr
Rb	Sr	Y	Zr	Nb	Mo	Tc	Ru	Rh	Pd	Ag	Cd	In	Sn	Sb	Te	I	Xe
Cs	Ba	La*	Hf	Ta	W	Re	Os	Ir	Pt	Au	Hg	Tl	Pb	Bi	Po	At	Rn
Fr	Ra	Ac**	104														

*LANTHANIDES	La	Ce	Pr	Nd	Pm	Sm	Eu	Gd	Tb	Dy	Ho	Er	Tm	Yb	Lu
**ACTINIDES	Ac	Th	Pa	U	Np	Pu	Am	Cm	Bk	Cf	Es	Fm	Md	102	Lw

Fig. 2-2.—The periodic chart of the elements. Elements in the same column have the same electronic structure in their outermost orbits and display similar chemical behavior.

up to the element number 105, which has 105 electrons. In Bohr's relatively simple model, the electrons are arranged in shells around the nucleus. Each shell has a letter designation: the innermost shell is called the K-shell and may contain one or two electrons. The next shell is known as the L-shell; it is further from the nucleus and may contain up to eight electrons. The next shell is called the M-shell and may contain up to 18 electrons. The letter designations for the other shells and their capacities are given in Table 2-1.

Sketches depicting the Bohr models of the first 20 elements are shown in Figure 2-3. The similarity in the electronic structures of lithium (Li), sodium (Na) and potassium (K) are obvious. Each of these three elements has one electron in the outermost shell. Lithium, sodium and potassium (as well as the heavier elements cesium and francium) are chemically

TABLE 2-1.—ATOMIC ELECTRON SHELLS AND THEIR CAPACITIES

SHELL LETTER DESIGNATION	TOTAL ELECTRON CAPACITY	CUMULATIVE TOTAL OF ELECTRONS
K	2	2
L	8	10
M	18	28
N	32	60
O	50	110
P	72	182

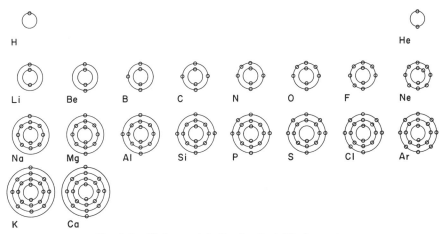

Fig. 2-3. — Bohr models for the first 20 elements.

very similar: they are all very reactive metals and can liberate hydrogen from water, all form soluble chloride and nitrate salts, and all have a chemical valence of one. (The concept of valence will not be discussed in detail here; it is sufficient to note that the valence is derived from the number of electrons in the outermost shell).

In a similar manner, the elements magnesium, calcium, barium, strontium and radium, all of which have two electrons in their outermost shells, would be expected to behave alike chemically. This is the basis for the use of strontium and barium isotopes in bone scanning (see Chap. 8). Since there are no physically attractive calcium isotopes, barium and strontium isotopes are used to detect bone lesions. Even in a chemically complex system such as the human body, these elements behave in similar fashion, and barium and strontium take the place of the calcium in bone mineral.

Elements which have the same electronic structures are arranged in the columns of the periodic chart shown in Figure 2-2. All the members of a given column have the same general chemical reactivity.

Atomic Structure and X-Rays

The radiation known as x-rays is a result of the movement of electrons from one shell to another. In x-ray tubes and in several radioactive decay processes, one or more electrons may be removed from the shells around the nucleus, creating a vacancy or hole. Energy is required to remove the electrons. In an x-ray tube, the energy is supplied by a high-speed beam of electrons striking the target anode. In radioactive elements, the energy is supplied by the decay process itself.

TABLE 2-2.— BINDING ENERGIES OF ELECTRONS IN VARIOUS
SHELLS OF ELEMENTS OF INTEREST IN NUCLEAR MEDICINE

ELEMENT	ATOMIC NUMBER	ELECTRON-BINDING ENERGY IN keV		
		K-shell	L-shell	M-shell
Fluorine	9	0.69	0.03	—
Sodium	11	1.07	0.06	—
Phosphorus	15	2.15	0.19	0.01
Gallium	31	10.37	1.30	0.16
Selenium	34	12.66	1.65	0.23
Rubidium	37	15.20	2.06	0.32
Strontium	38	16.10	2.22	0.36
Technetium	43	21.04	3.04	0.54
Indium	49	27.94	4.24	0.83
Iodine	53	33.17	5.19	1.07
Xenon	54	34.56	5.45	1.14
Gold	79	80.72	14.35	3.42
Mercury	80	83.10	14.84	3.56

The energy required to remove an electron from an atom depends on the element and on the shell from which it is removed. The minimum quantity of energy necessary is called the shell-binding energy. The values for the binding energies of electrons in shells of several elements of interest in nuclear medicine are given in Table 2-2. Note that the electron-binding energy increases with atomic number for each shell.

As mentioned earlier, x-rays arise when an electron moves from one shell to another. The energy of the emitted x-ray is equal to the difference between the electron-binding energies of the shells. Thus the x-ray emitted when an electron moves from the L-shell to the K-shell in an iodine atom is 29 kiloelectron volts. Remember that a vacancy in a shell (a process that requires at least the binding energy of the shell) must be created first. Since the electron-binding energy increases with atomic number, the energy of the emitted x-ray also increases with atomic number. The x-radiation emitted when an electron moves from L, M, N,

Fig. 2-4. — Production of K-characteristic x-rays in an atom.

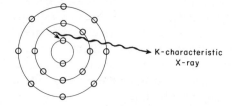

VACANCY CREATED
IN
ELECTRON INNERSHELL

VACANCY FILLED BY ELECTRON
MOVING FROM OUTER SHELL,
PRODUCING X-RAY

K-characteristic
X-ray

TABLE 2-3.—CHARACTERISTIC X-RAYS FOR SEVERAL ELEMENTS

ELEMENT	ATOMIC NUMBER	CHARACTERISTIC K X-RAY ENERGY (keV)
Selenium	34	11.2
Technetium	43	18.4
Iodine	53	28.6
Xenon	54	29.8
Mercury	80	70.8

etc. shell to the K-shell is called the K-characteristic x-ray, characteristic because it is unique to each element. The process is shown schematically in Figure 2-4.

Similarly, when an electron moves from an M, N, O, *etc.* shell to a vacancy in the L-shell, an L-characteristic x-ray is emitted. Characteristic x-rays for several elements are listed in Table 2-3. These characteristic x-rays are sometimes used for nuclear medicine studies. For example, the K-characteristic x-rays of iodine 125 and mercury 197 are used routinely for thyroid evaluation and kidney scanning, respectively.

The Bohr Atom and the Quantum-Mechanical Atom

The Bohr atomic model assigns the negatively charged electrons to orbits which revolve around the nucleus. Bohr's contribution to atomic physics was his contention that the electrons could occupy orbits of fixed radius only (the process is called quantization). The equation giving the orbital radius is:

$$r = \frac{Cn^2}{Z} \tag{2-1}$$

in which r is the orbital radius, C is a constant, Z is the atomic number, and n is a number which can have only integral values (1, 2, 3, *etc.*). The value of n is also known as the principal quantum number. Three other quantum numbers have been proposed to describe completely the behavior of atomic electrons; 1, the secondary quantum number, m, the magnetic quantum number, and s, the spin quantum number. Each quantum number is associated with a definite electronic state. A change in quantum number is accompanied by the absorption or emission of a definite amount of energy by the atom.

As mentioned in the preceding section, the electrons surrounding the nucleus are arranged according to a rigid set of rules which permit 2 electrons in the first orbit, 8 electrons in the second, 18 in the third, *etc.* The arrangement of electrons in the orbits is the determining factor in the chemical behavior of an element.

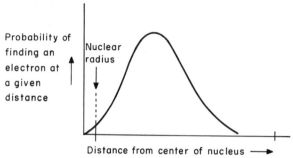

Fig. 2-5.—One solution to the quantum-mechanical equations for the hydrogen atom. The probability of finding an electron at any given distance from the center of the nucleus is plotted as a function of that distance.

Because of limitations of the Bohr model (important examples will be discussed in later chapters), the wave-mechanical model of the atom has been developed. Instead of assigning a particular radius to an orbital electron, the solution of a quantum-mechanical equation provides an estimate of the probability of finding an electron in the region around the nucleus. A graph of the solution is shown in Figure 2-5 for the hydrogen atom electron. Translated into a model, the hydrogen atom electron is now represented as a spherical cloud of negative charge around the nucleus.

A number of interesting points can be established from Figure 2-5: (1) the most likely place to find the electron is at distance r, which is exactly the Bohr radius for the hydrogen atom electron; (2) the probability surface is spherical, rather than circular, as were the Bohr orbits; (3) there is a finite probability of finding the electron within the nucleus.

Atomic Weights and Isotopes

Since individual atoms weigh only a small fraction of a gram—approximately 10^{-22} grams—a relative scale of atomic weights has been developed. The weight of an atom is compared to the weight of the most common isotope of carbon, carbon 12, which is assigned a weight of 12.0000 atomic mass units (amu). On this scale, hydrogen atoms weigh one amu, fluorine atoms weigh 19 amu and iodine atoms, 127 amu. The constituents of the nucleus, the proton and the neutron, each weigh one amu.

If a sample of the metal tin (50 protons) were examined with a mass spectrometer, tin atoms weighing between 112 and 124 amu would be observed. Since each of these atoms must contain only 50 protons, the mass differences must be accounted for by differences in the number of neutrons. The nucleus which weighs 112 amu must contain 62 neutrons (called N, the neutron number). The sum of the number of protons and number of neutrons is the mass number (A). The hypothetic element Q, with mass number A, proton number Z and neutron number N is written in shorthand:

$$^A_Z Q_N.$$

Thus, tin-112 is denoted by $^{112}_{50}Sn_{62}$, which contains a number of redundancies. Most often, tin-112 would be written simply as ^{112}Sn.

Atoms with the same proton number Z but with different neutron numbers (N) are called isotopes. Isotopes are identified by their element name and mass number; for example ^{113}Sn, ^{99m}Tc.

The Nucleus and Level Schemes

Although the nucleus has never been seen, models of the nucleus have been constructed which are based on a large body of experimental data. Physicists use models to help them visualize what the nucleus looks like and to predict the outcome of future experiments. Just as in the case of the electronic structure of the atom, there are a number of nuclear models which are useful in understanding the nucleus. Two of the most popular models are the shell model and the liquid-drop model. In the shell model, protons and neutrons are said to be arranged in shells inside the nucleus, much like the electrons outside the nucleus. According to this model, the properties of any given nucleus are dependent chiefly on the outermost nucleons. In the liquid-drop model, the nucleus is considered to be like a drop of water with the ability to be deformed and split, as in the process of fission.

Whatever nuclear model is used, a nucleus can be said to exist in a

Fig. 2-6. – Nuclear level scheme for ^{99m}Tc.

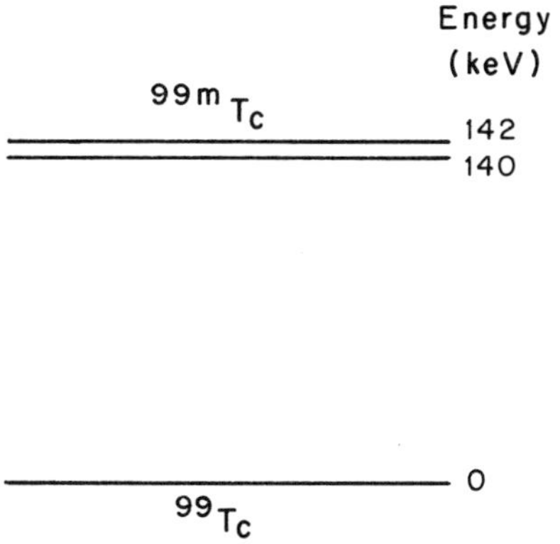

number of discrete energy states or levels. These energy levels are usually depicted as horizontal lines in nuclear level schemes. The lowest energy state of any nucleus is called the ground state. Levels with more energy than the ground state are called excited states. The nuclear level scheme for ^{99}Tc (43 protons, 56 neutrons) is shown in Figure 2-6. The bottom line is the ground state and is assigned zero energy; this state has the lowest energy of all the possible arrangements of 43 protons and 56 neutrons. The line identified as 140 keV is the first excited state; this level has more energy (140 keV more) than the ground state and it represents a different configuration of the 43 protons and 56 neutrons. The shell model would say that the forty-third proton was in a different shell. The 142-keV line in Figure 2-5 is the second excited state, with a third, more energetic configuration of the 43 protons and 56 neutrons. This particular energy level is of particular importance to nuclear medicine, since it is known as ^{99m}Tc and is relatively stable.

The important points to remember are that each energy level consists of a particular configuration of protons and neutrons, and that only discrete energy levels exist for the nucleus—for example, the only low-energy states of ^{99}Tc are at 0, 140 and 142 keV.

SUGGESTED READING

Blahd, W. H. (ed.) *Nuclear Medicine* (2d ed.; New York: McGraw-Hill Book Company, Inc., 1971), Chap. 1.

Friedlander, G., Kennedy, J. W., and Miller, J. M.: *Nuclear and Radiochemistry* (2d ed.; New York: John Wiley and Sons, Inc., 1964), Chap. 2.

Lederer, C. M., Hollander, J. M., and Perlman, I.: *Table of Isotopes* (6th ed.; New York: John Wiley and Sons, Inc., 1967).

Glasstone, S: Sourcebook on Atomic Energy (New York: D. Van Nostrand Co., Inc., 1950), Chaps. 1, 2, 4.

STUDY QUESTIONS

1. Name the three basic constituents of atoms and give their relative weights.
2. What are the advantages and disadvantages of the Bohr model of the atom?
3. What other possible models had been proposed before Bohr?
4. How is a sodium atom different from a cesium atom, and in what ways are they the same?
5. Element 110 may be among the very heaviest stable elements. To what element would you expect its chemical behavior to be similar?
6. Explain how K-characteristic x-rays are produced.
7. What is the binding energy of an electron?
8. How does the quantum-mechanical model of the atom differ from the Bohr model?
9. What element has the most isotopes?
10. Draw the nuclear level schemes for the decay of the following radioisotopes: ^{113m}In, ^{125}I, ^{18}F, ^{137}Cs and ^{203}Hg.

CHAPTER 3

Electromagnetic Radiation

ALMOST ALL DIAGNOSTIC STUDIES performed in nuclear medicine involve the counting of gamma rays, a form of electromagnetic radiation. Since this radiation is central to so many aspects of nuclear medicine, it is important to understand what electromagnetic radiation is.

Wavelength and Frequency

Electromagnetic radiation is a term applied to a particular class of wave motions involving waves which have associated with them oscillating electric and magnetic fields which are perpendicular to each other and to the direction of propagation of the wave. In these terms, a single light ray can be represented as in Figure 3-1. In this figure, the electric field of the ray oscillates in the plane of the paper, the magnetic field moves in and out of the paper perpendicular to the plane of the paper, and the ray moves from left to right, as indicated by the arrow.

For clarity, a ray of electromagnetic radiation is usually represented as a single oscillating field, as shown in Figure 3-2. All electromagnetic radiations travel at the speed of light $- 3 \times 10^{10}$cm./sec. in a vacuum. An electromagnetic wave may be characterized by two properties: its wavelength (λ in Figure 3-2) and its amplitude (Fig. 3-2). The wavelength is the distance between any two corresponding points on the oscillating curve. The wavelength is usually designated by the Greek letter lambda

Fig. 3-1. — An electromagnetic wave. The electric and magnetic fields oscillate at right angles to each other and to the direction of propagation.

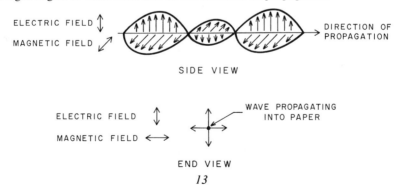

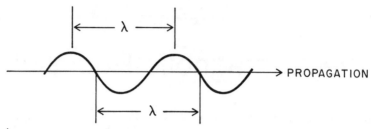

λ = ONE WAVELENGTH

Fig. 3-2. — A simplified sketch of an electromagnetic wave. The wavelength is the distance between any two successive peaks.

(λ). Another term that is often used to describe electromagnetic radiation is the frequency, which is the number of oscillations that the electric field undergoes per second. The frequency is usually denoted by the Greek letter nu (ν). Recently, a new unit has been approved for denoting frequency — the hertz, abbreviated hz, which is one cycle per second. Frequency and wavelength are inversely proportional to each other. The proportionality constant is c, the speed of light, or 3×10^{10} cm./sec. The relationship between wavelength, frequency and the speed of light is given in the following equation:

$$\lambda \nu = c. \tag{3-1}$$

This equation can be used to determine the frequency of an electromagnetic wave, if its wavelength is known, by rearranging equation 3-1 to read

$$\nu = \frac{c}{\lambda}. \tag{3-2}$$

In a similar manner, the wavelength of a wave of given frequency is calculated by

$$\lambda = \frac{c}{\nu}. \tag{3-3}$$

Another way of describing an electromagnetic wave is to state its energy, usually in electron volts (ev) or some multiple of ev, such as kiloelectron volts (keV) or megaelectron volts (MeV). The energy (E) of an electromagnetic wave is related to its frequency as follows:

$$E(ev) = (4.13 \times 10^{21})\nu(hz). \tag{3-4}$$

Using equation (3-2), the energy may also be calculated from the wavelength:

$$E(ev) = \frac{1.24 \times 10^{-4}}{\lambda(cm.)}. \tag{3-5}$$

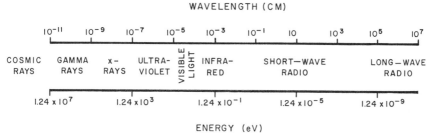

WAVELENGTH (CM)

Fig. 3-3. — The electromagnetic spectrum, which stretches from the radio wavelengths, through visible light and into the cosmic ray region.

The Electromagnetic Spectrum

The name applied to electromagnetic radiation depends on its wavelength. Figure 3-3 illustrates the electromagnetic spectrum and the names associated with different wavelengths. Several points should be noted in Figure 3-3. Energy and frequency decrease from left to right, and wavelength increases in the same direction. The boundaries between most adjacent regions are not sharp. The x-ray spectrum overlaps the gamma ray region. The figure is indicative of the importance of electromagnetic radiation in everyday life, with the spectrum stretching from cosmic rays to long- and short-wave radio and television. The narrow region of the electromagnetic spectrum between the wavelengths 4,000 and 8,000 Angströms is what human beings call visible light. It is interesting to note that the spectrum of the electromagnetic radiation reaching the earth's surface from the sun is also in this region. Thus, the evolutionary processes which brought about human color vision were guided by the main light source illuminating the planet. If vision has developed in planetary systems near x-ray stars, presumably it would be termed x-ray vision by earth's standard.

Electromagnetic radiation is produced when electric charges move. Visible light arises from moderate excitation of atomic electrons, such as occurs in an incandescent bulb. Gamma rays arise from the atomic nucleus during a rearrangement of charges in the nucleus. As mentioned in Chapter 2, characteristic x-rays are produced when an electron moves from a higher atomic shell to a lower shell.

Mass and Energy

The concept of the equivalency of mass and energy is part of one of the most basic sets of laws of physics — the conservation laws. Simply stated,

TABLE 3-1.—MASS AND ENERGY EQUIVALENTS

CONVERSION PROCESS	MASS EQUIVALENT Grams	ENERGY EQUIVALENT Calories
One 1.00 MeV gamma ray	1.86×10^{-27}	3.84×10^{-14}
Creation of electron-positron pair	1.90×10^{-27}	3.92×10^{-14}
Complete decay of 10 millicuries of ^{99m}Tc to ^{99}Tc	2.92×10^{-15}	0.0628
500 rads whole-body radiation	3.89×10^{-12}	80.1
Complete combustion of one gallon of gasoline in air	1.96×10^{-6}	4.04×10^{7}
Nuclear fission of 1.00 Gm. of ^{235}U	9.13×10^{-4}	1.88×10^{10}
Nuclear fusion 1.00 Gm. H converted to 1.00 Gm. He	7.18×10^{-3}	1.48×10^{11}
20 kilotons of TNT explosion	0.985	2.00×10^{13}
One gram of any material object converted to energy	1.00	2.06×10^{13}
2 megatons of TNT explosion	98.5	2.00×10^{15}

it is a law that energy cannot be created or destroyed, but can only be converted from one form to another. Einstein's famous equation is an expression of that law:

$$E = mc^2. \tag{3-6}$$

Here, E is the amount of energy (in ergs) which can be obtained from a mass m (in grams), and c is the velocity of light in a vacuum, 3.0×10^{10} cm./sec. The equation states that energy can be obtained from material objects; what is not generally recognized is that it is possible to obtain material objects from energy. If enough energy is provided, for example, in the form of a gamma ray, it is possible to produce two electrons (see Chap. 6).

To provide the reader with some "feel" for mass-energy relationship, Table 3-1 lists the mass and energy equivalents for a number of conversions. As indicated in the table, the 20 kiloton nuclear weapon which essentially destroyed the city of Hiroshima, Japan, involved the conversion of only one gram of mass into energy. On the other end of the energy scale, a 1.00 MeV gamma ray is equivalent to the conversion of 1.86×10^{-27} Gm. of matter. In a more familiar example, the complete combustion of one gallon of gasoline, producing about 40 million calories, involves the transformation of about 2 μg. of gasoline into energy.

SUGGESTED READING

Glasstone, S.: *Sourcebook on Atomic Energy* (New York: D. Van Nostrand Co., Inc., 1950), Chap. 3.

Johns, H. E.: *The Physics of Radiology* (2d ed.; Springfield, Ill.: Charles C Thomas, Publisher, 1964).

STUDY QUESTIONS

1. How does an electromagnetic wave differ from other waves, such as sound waves and water waves?
2. How are the wavelength and frequency of an electromagnetic wave related?
3. Calculate the missing quantities in the table below:

Wavelength	Frequency	Energy
4,000 Angströms		
12,000 Angströms		
		140 keV
		364 keV
	1,300 kilohertz	
	100 megahertz	
	60 hertz	
1.0 Angström		
		25 keV
		1.17 keV
		75 keV
	1.0 hertz	
550 Angströms		
		1.0 ev

CHAPTER 4

Electrostatics

ELECTROSTATICS IS A BRANCH OF PHYSICS that deals with static electric charges. The science of electrostatics touches many areas of nuclear physics, and it is important that the student become familiar with the laws of electrostatics and their applications to nuclear medicine.

Introduction to Static Charge

Static electric charges arise when electrons are transferred from one object to another. An object having an excess of electrons is said to have a negative (−) charge, whereas objects with a deficiency of electrons are called positively (+) charged. Static charges can be obtained by a number of methods, the most familiar of which is friction. When a person walks across a nylon carpet in a relatively dry room, electrons are wiped off the carpet onto his shoes; the walker then acquires a negative charge. The excess electrons are released in the form of a spark when the charged person approaches a grounded object.

As mentioned in Chapter 2, each electron has one negative charge and is the basic unit of electricity. In electrostatic units (esu), the charge on each electron is 4.80×10^{-10} esu. Since this is an extremely small amount of charge, a more practical system is usually used when describing charge. In this system the coulomb is the basic unit of charge, and consists of the charge associated with 6.24×10^{18} electrons.

Although it is possible to charge an object by adding or removing electrons, the over-all net charge in the universe is believed to be zero. Thus, the creation of a positively-charged object implies that there is also a negatively-charged body in order that an electrically neutral universe be maintained. This is another of the conservation laws of physics in action: charge, like mass and energy, cannot be created or destroyed.

The Laws of Electrostatics

The first two laws of electrostatics are simple: like charges repel each other, unlike charges attract. The attractive (or repulsive) force is directly proportional to the charge on each object and inversely proportional to the square of the distance between them. The equation which describes the force is known as Coulomb's law and is expressed as follows:

$$F = \frac{Kq_1q_2}{d^2}.$$ (4-1)

Here, F is the force exerted on each object, q_1 and q_2 are the charges on each object, and d is the distance between them.

Electrostatic forces are used to accelerate electrons in x-ray tubes. Electrons are boiled off a hot filament and attracted toward a positively charged anode. The electrostatic forces are also employed in a number of detection systems used in nuclear medicine (see Chap. 7).

The Electron Volt

The amount of charge on an object can be determined by measuring the work required to move a second object carrying charge of the same sign toward the first. The amount of work necessary is synonymous with the energy expended in moving the charge. This brings us to an important definition in electrostatics: the work, or energy, or potential difference in an electrostatic system. The unit is the volt, a familiar electric term. The fact that the volt is a measure of the energy of a system is stressed here, because many of the energy quantities in nuclear medicine are measured in volts. The formal definition of a volt is as follows: one volt is the potential difference between two points such that one joule of work must be performed in order to move one coulomb of charge between the two points. (A joule is equivalent to 0.239 calories and is the amount of work required to lift one pound about nine inches off the ground.)

In nuclear medicine, the electron volt (ev) is a more useful term. One ev is the energy acquired by an electron when it falls through a potential difference of one volt. The process is illustrated in Figure 4-1. The distance between the potential points is not material. One electron volt is the energy acquired by the electron no matter what distance separates the two points. Since the electron weighs only 9.1 × 10⁻²⁸ Gm. and its velocity after traveling between a potential difference of one volt is 5.92 × 10⁷ cm./sec., its kinetic energy can be calculated from the equation

$$E = 1/2\ mv^2.$$ (4-2)

In equation 4-2, the energy comes out in ergs if the mass is given in grams and the velocity is expressed in centimeters per second. Substituting the values just mentioned for the electron's mass and energy, the energy is found to be 1.60 × 10⁻¹² erg, which is equivalent to one ev. One erg is about the energy deposited by a fly hitting a brick wall at top

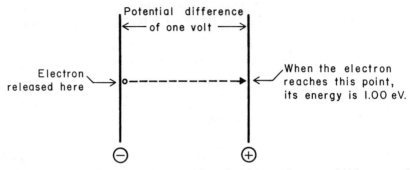

Fig. 4-1.—The electron volt (ev). After the electron has traveled between the two plates, its energy is one ev. The distance separating the plates is immaterial.

speed. Since an electron volt is only about one trillionth of an erg, it is apparent that an electron volt is an extremely small quantity of energy. Table 4-1 gives the energy equivalents of some familiar (and not so familiar) energy terms used in physics and nuclear medicine. Note that 1,000 ev is called the kiloelectron volt (keV) and one million ev is denoted as MeV (megaelectron volt), and these are still relatively small amounts of energy.

A clear distinction should be made between the potential (voltage) and the energy (electron volts) of a system. The center wire of a Geiger-Müller (G-M) tube may have a potential of approximately +1,000 volts, relative to zero volts or ground potential. When radiation interacts with the gas in the G-M tube and creates positive ions and electrons, the electrons are attracted toward the center wire. The electrons acquire energy as they are moved.

TABLE 4-1.—ENERGY EQUIVALENTS OF FAMILIAR AND UNFAMILIAR
PHYSICAL UNITS

ENERGY EQUIVALENT OF ELECTRON	ELECTRON VOLT	ERG	JOULE	CALORIE	B.T.U.	WATT-HOUR
1.00 volt (ev)	1	1.6×10^{-12}	1.6×10^{-19}	3.8×10^{-20}	1.5×10^{-22}	4.7×10^{-23}
1.00 keV	1×10^3	1.6×10^{-9}	1.6×10^{-16}	3.8×10^{-17}	1.5×10^{-19}	4.7×10^{-20}
1.00 MeV	1×10^6	1.6×10^{-6}	1.6×10^{-13}	3.8×10^{-14}	1.5×10^{-16}	4.7×10^{-17}
1.00 Erg	6.2×10^{11}	1	1.0×10^{-7}	2.39×10^{-8}	9.5×10^{-10}	2.9×10^{-11}
1.00 Joule	6.2×10^{18}	1.0×10^7	1	0.239	9.5×10^{-3}	2.8×10^{-4}
1.00 Calorie	2.6×10^{19}	4.2×10^7	4.18	1	4.0×10^{-3}	1.2×10^{-3}
1.00 B.T.U.	6.2×10^{21}	1.0×10^{10}	1.0×10^3	2.52×10^2	1	0.31
1.00 Watt-hour	2.1×10^{22}	3.4×10^{10}	3.4×10^3	8.6×10^2	3.41	1
1.00 Gm. matter	5.6×10^{32}	9.0×10^{20}	9.0×10^{13}	2.3×10^{13}	9.0×10^{10}	2.6×10^{10}

Power Supplies

Although it is possible to develop a fairly large potential difference by walking across a nylon carpet in a relatively dry room, this method turns out to be very inconvenient for producing potential differences in nuclear detectors. Almost all detection systems used in nuclear medicine require a source of high voltage, or potential (see Chap. 7). Voltages of up to about 1,500 volts are common in most scanning and camera systems; these voltages are provided by a unit which is usually termed the power supply.

TRANSFORMERS

Power supplies convert the 110-volt alternating current (AC) obtained from a wall outlet to a direct current (DC) voltage of up to 1,500 volts. In battery-operated devices such as portable survey meters, the few-volt DC output of the battery pack is converted to a DC voltage of about 1,000 volts. In the 110-volt AC system, the 110-volt output is stepped up to 1,500 volts by using a transformer, as indicated in Figure 4-2. The AC voltage on the secondary side of the transformer depends on the number of turns on the secondary side. In mathematic form, the secondary voltage (V_2) is given by

$$V_2 = \frac{T_2}{T_1} V_1 \qquad (4\text{-}3)$$

in which T_2 and T_1 are the number of terms on the secondary and primary side of the transformer, respectively, and V_1 is the AC voltage applied to the primary coil.

Note that in Figure 4-2 the number of turns on the secondary side can

Fig. 4-2.—A step-up transformer. There are more windings on the secondary than on the primary side. A selection switch is provided to produce various AC output voltage.

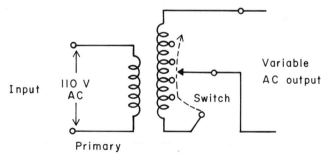

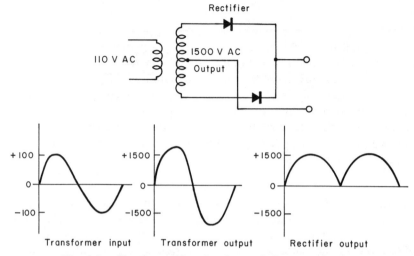

Fig. 4-3. — Simple rectifier circuit coupled to transformer.

be changed by moving the switch. In this way the secondary, or high, voltage can be varied. The input and output voltages of the transformer are both AC, which is the only type on which transformers operate.

RECTIFIERS AND FILTERS

Rectifiers convert the high-voltage alternating current of the transformer's secondary portion to direct current. A simple rectifier system is shown in Figure 4-3. The rectifier circuit functions through the circuit components (indicated in the figure by the symbol →►-) which allow current to flow in only one direction. These components are called diodes and may be either tube or solid-state devices.

The output of the rectifier circuit is still not suitable for use in detection

Fig. 4-4. — Simple filter circuit coupled to transformer for smoothing DC voltage.

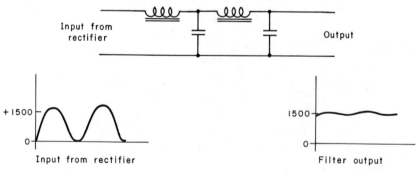

systems, however, since, as indicated in Figure 4-3, the voltage still shows considerable variation with time. In order to smooth out the DC voltage of the rectifier, a filter is used. A simple filter consisting of two inductance coils and two capacitors in the circuit is shown in Figure 4-4. The variation in the DC voltage has been reduced to a slight ripple. Much more sophisticated circuits are used in most power supplies available commercially, with the ripple, or variation, in the DC voltage output usually being of the order of one volt or less at 1,000 volts output. This precision is required in order that the characteristics of detectors not change during the time that several nuclear radiation events are being detected.

BATTERY-OPERATED POWER SUPPLIES

Battery-operated instruments, such as survey meters and ionization chambers, also require a source of DC high voltage. The batteries provide a DC voltage, but usually of 9 volts or less. The problem is to increase the DC voltage to 1,000 volts or more. Since transformers operate only on alternating current, the DC output of the batteries is first converted to AC. The conversion may be simply a mechanical device which makes and breaks a circuit or, more usually, an electronic system which accomplishes the same thing. After conversion to AC, the rest of the system for producing high-voltage DC is just as previously described for power supplies operating on 100 volts AC from a wall outlet.

The applications of electrostatics and power supplies to nuclear medicine will be discussed in detail in Chapter 6.

SUGGESTED READING

Selman, J.: *The Fundamentals of X-Ray and Radium Physics* (4th ed.; Springfield, Ill.: Charles C Thomas, Publisher, 1965), Chaps. 5, 10, 11.

STUDY QUESTIONS

1. Describe the difference between positively and negatively charged objects.
2. The force of repulsion between two charged objects 2 inches apart is 10 dynes. What is the force between the same objects when they are separated by 3 inches?
3. Explain the difference between one kilovolt (kv) and one kiloelectron volt (keV).
4. What is the chief use of high-voltage power supplies in nuclear medicine instrumentation?

CHAPTER 5

Radioactivity

RADIOACTIVITY WAS DISCOVERED by Becquerel in 1897, and in the seventy-odd years since its discovery it has been one of the central experimental facts of nuclear physics. Radioactive isotopes are still being discovered, although at a much slower rate than in the 1940s and 1950s. The process of radioactive decay is absolutely required for nuclear medicine studies. Every in vivo and in vitro test performed in nuclear medicine depends on radioactive decay and the detection of the radiations emitted in decay.

The Half Life

When an isotope is said to be radioactive, this means that the nuclei of the atoms of that isotope are undergoing spontaneous disintegration. Obviously, all the nuclei do not disintegrate at once, nor do they all last forever. One of the earliest discoveries made concerning radioactive materials was that each radioisotope undergoes decay with a definite half period, or half life. For example, the radiations from ^{210}Po were found to diminish to one half of their initial intensity in about 140 days. The half life of a radioactive material is defined as the time required for the activity to decrease to one half of its initial value.

Half lives of radioactive nuclides range from fractions of a second to billions of years. Tables giving the half lives of radionuclides as well as other properties are available from the General Electric Company, Schenectady, New York. The half life of any radioactive nuclide is a physical characteristic of that nuclide and cannot be changed by any physical or chemical reaction. Thus, the half life of ^{131}I is 8.05 days, whether it is in a bottle as sodium iodide at 0 C., in the thyroid gland of a human being as thyroid hormone at 38 C., or in the middle of the sun at several million degrees centigrade.

Half lives of radioactive materials are usually determined by measuring the amount of activity in a sample over a period of time. The results of a hypothetic experiment performed with ^{131}I are given in Table 5-1. The experimental data are also plotted in Figure 5-1. By drawing a smooth curve through the data, it is possible to determine that the activity decreases by one half in 8 days. A much more valuable graph of the ex-

TABLE 5-1.—RESULTS OF A COUNTING EXPERIMENT DESIGNED
TO DETERMINE THE HALF LIFE OF ^{131}I

DAY OF COUNT	SAMPLE COUNTS PER MINUTE
0	15,000
1	13,700
2	12,600
3	11,600
4	10,650
7	8,200
8	7,550
10	6,350
15	4,130
18	3,180
21	2,460
25	1,740
30	1,140

perimental data can be obtained by plotting the results on a semilog graph
— one in which the activity is plotted on a logarithmic scale against time
on a linear scale, as shown in Figure 5-2. Here, it can be seen that the
results produce a straight line, from which it is very easy to determine the
half-life. Following the straight line on the graph of Figure 5-2 between
any two points which are related by a factor of one-half will indicate the

Fig. 5-1.— The decay of a sample of ^{131}I, from data in Table 5 – 1. Both ordinate
abscissa of this graph have linear scales. Compare with Figure 5 – 2.

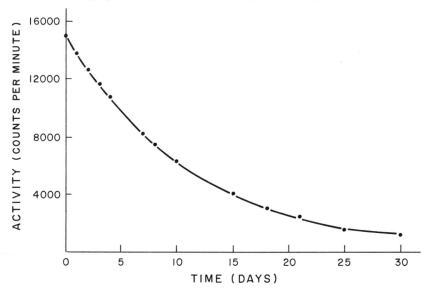

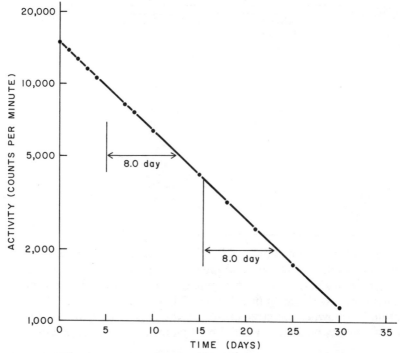

Fig. 5-2. — The decay of a sample of ^{131}I, from data in Table 5 – 1. The ordinate (activity scale) of this graph is logarithmic, whereas the time scale is linear. Compare with Figure 5 – 1.

half life. Since the half life of an isotope is a constant characteristic of that isotope, the determination of the half life can be a very important clue in identifying an unknown isotope.

Units of Radioactivity

Radioactivity in nuclear medicine is usually measured in units of curies (Ci), millicuries (mCi), or microcuries (μCi). The curie was originally defined in terms of the number of disintegrations per second of one gram

TABLE 5-2. — DEFINITIONS OF THE CURIE
AND ITS SUBUNITS

UNIT	ABBREVIATION	DISINTEGRATIONS PER SECOND	DISINTEGRATIONS PER MINUTE
Curie	Ci	3.70×10^{10}	2.22×10^{12}
Millicurie	mCi	3.70×10^{7}	2.22×10^{9}
Microcurie	μCi	3.70×10^{4}	2.22×10^{6}
Nanocurie	nCi	3.70×10^{1}	2.22×10^{3}

of ^{226}Ra, but is now defined as 3.70×10^{10} (37 billion) disintegrations per second of any radioactive material. Table 5-2 lists the disintegration rates for the quantities mentioned above. Note that the curie and its subunits are defined in terms of disintegration per unit time, and *not* in counts per unit time.

Calculations Involving the Half Life

The amount of radioactivity contained in a sample provided by a pharmaceutical manufacturer is usually specified as to date. For example, a sample of ^{131}I may have a label stating its activity to be 140 mCi in 10 ml. of solution on October 1. The technician's problem is that it is now October 13 and a patient is waiting to receive a therapeutic dose of 5 mCi of ^{131}I. The problem is usually solved by looking at a decay chart provided by one of the drug manufacturers, but it is possible to do the calculation yourself.

Numerically, the amount of activity remaining in a sample of radioactive material after time t is given by

$$A = A_0 \, e^{-\frac{0.693\, t}{t_{1/2}}} \qquad (5\text{-}1)$$

in which A is the activity remaining at time t,

A_0 is the initial activity,

$t_{1/2}$ is the half life of the radioactive material, and

e is the base of the natural logarithmic scale.

Although equation 5-1 can appear rather formidable to a technician who has forgotten almost all the mathematics he ever knew, the equation can be considerably simplified. First, we rearrange equation 5-1 slightly to read

$$\frac{A}{A_0} = e^{-\frac{0.693\, t}{t_{1/2}}} \qquad (5\text{-}2)$$

in which the quantity on the left is the fraction of the initial activity remaining. The equation may now be converted to logarithmic form, as follows:

$$\log_{10}\left(\frac{A}{A_0}\right) = \frac{-0.300\, t}{t_{1/2}}. \qquad (5\text{-}3)$$

Using the data given in the problem above (the half life of ^{131}I is 8.05 days), equation (5-3) now reads

$$\log_{10}\left(\frac{A}{A_0}\right) = \frac{-0.300 \times 12}{8.05}$$

$$= -0.447$$

$$\log_{10}\left(\frac{A}{A_o}\right) = 9.553 - 10.$$

At this point, it might be useful for the reader to review the section on logarithms in Appendix B. Continuing with the problem, we find $A/A_o = 0.356$; that is, 35.6% of the initial activity remains. Thus the activity remaining on October 13 is 50.0 mCi in 10 ml. of solution, and the waiting patient should receive 1.0 ml. of solution.

In many cases, manufacturers predate their radiopharmaceuticals, so that it is necessary to determine the activity before the calibration date. In the previous example, it may be September 20, and a dose of 5 mCi is required. Equation 5-3 is used again, but here the t is entered as a negative number:

$$\log_{10}\left(\frac{A}{A_o}\right) = \frac{-0.300 \times (-11)}{8.05}$$

$$\log_{10}\left(\frac{A}{A_o}\right) = +0.409.$$

Looking up the log in a table, we find $A/A_o = 2.560$, that is, the activity on September 20 is 2.560 times the activity on October 1, or 358 mCi in 10 ml. and the patient should receive 0.140 milliliters of solution.

Specific Activity

Specific activity is a confusing term because it is used to define several different quantities. In most cases in nuclear medicine, the term refers to the number of millicuries per milliliter (mCi/ml.) of solution in a sample. For example, a sample of ^{99m}Tc may have a specific activity of 10.5 mCi/ml. at 9:00 A.M. on December 1. Decay calculations involving the specific activity are done exactly as outlined in the previous section. Thus, at 3:00 P.M. on December 1 (one half life later), the ^{99m}Tc sample mentioned above will have a specific activity of 5.25 mCi/ml.

The second type of specific activity refers to the activity (curies, millicuries) per unit weight (gram, milligram, *etc.*). This definition of specific activity is important also, since it gives an indication of how much material is associated with the radioactivity involved in a study. First, consider a sample of radioactive material which contains *only* radioactive atoms, such as ^{99m}Tc. This sample is said to be carrier-free, that is, it contains no other technetium atoms except the radioactive ^{99m}Tc. Its specific activity is as high as possible. The weight of a sample of radioactive atoms is related to the activity of the sample, the atomic weight of the atoms, and the half life, as follows:

$$W = 3.18 \times 10^{-13}(A)(\text{At. Wt.})(t_{1/2}) \qquad (5\text{-}4)$$

in which W is the weight of the sample in grams,
A is the activity of the sample in mCi,
At. Wt. is the atomic weight of the atoms, and
$t_{1/2}$ is the half-life in hours.

The units (mCi for activity and hours for the half-life) must be correctly entered. Using the values for 1.0 mCi of ^{99m}Tc ($t_{1/2}$ = 6.0 hours, At. Wt. = 99), we have

$$W = 1.89 \times 10^{-10} \, \text{Gm.}$$

Thus, the specific activity of 1.00 mCi of ^{99m}Tc, in the carrier-free state, is 1.00 mCi per 1.89×10^{-10} Gm., or 5.30×10^6 (5.3 million) curies per gram!

Next, consider a carrier-free sample of ^{131}I containing 1.00 mCi of activity. Again using equation 5-4, we find the weight of 1.00 mCi of ^{131}I to be 8.06×10^{-9} gram, so the specific activity is 1.26×10^5 curies per gram. However, most samples of ^{131}I contain other iodine atoms, usually the stable isotope ^{127}I which is added during chemical processing of the material, so the isotope is rarely available in carrier-free form and its specific activity is usually much lower than indicated above.

A third type of sample is exemplified by the materials used for lung scanning: macroaggregated human serum albumin (MAA) which can be labeled with ^{131}I or ^{99m}Tc. In this case, the specific activity is usually quoted in terms of the amount of activity per unit weight of the labeled compound—for example, 2.5 mCi per milligram of MAA.

Natural and Artificial Radioactivity

The first radioactive element to be discovered was polonium, as the isotope ^{210}Po. Polonium, and all the elements heavier than bismuth, up to uranium, are radioactive and occur in nature. These radioactive nuclides, along with several others, are termed natural radioactivity, since they were apparently produced sometime before the formation of the solar system.

THE NATURALLY OCCURRING RADIOACTIVE SERIES

All of the isotopes of all the elements between polonium and uranium are radioactive. Three long-lived nuclides, ^{232}Th, ^{235}U and ^{238}U, are the sources of three series of radioactive isotopes. The three series exist today in nature by virtue of the long half lives of ^{232}Th, ^{235}U and ^{238}U. They simply have not had time to decay completely. Much of the work in radiation physics during the first 40 years of this century was devoted to working out the decay relationships among members of the three series. In fact, the final piece of the puzzle was not put in place until

1939, when Marguerite Perey discovered element number 87, francium.

The uranium (4n + 2) series. — Uranium-238, which makes up 99.3% of the uranium on the earth, has a half life of 4.5×10^9 years, and decays to ^{234}Th, which in turn decays with a half life of 24.1 days to ^{234}Pa, which is also radioactive. After 10 more decays, the final product of the series is ^{206}Pb, which is stable. Each of the isotopes in this series has a mass number which, when divided by four, leaves a remainder of two; thus, the series is called the 4n + 2 radioactive series. The complete uranium series is given in Table 5-3. This series includes ^{226}Ra, which was the second element to be discovered by virtue of its radioactivity and has been an important source of radiation in the radiotherapy for cancer.

In an undisturbed sample of uranium ore, each of the nuclides will be present in equilibrium with ^{238}U. This means that if the sample contains a millicurie of ^{238}U, there will also be a millicurie of each of the other members of the series. The concept of radioactive equilibrium is discussed in greater detail in a later section.

The series terminates with a stable isotope of lead, ^{206}Pb. It is possible to estimate the age of a uranium ore sample by determining the amount of ^{206}Pb in the sample relative to other stable lead isotopes and to the amount of ^{238}U and ^{235}U.

The actinium (4n + 3) series. — This series begins with ^{235}U, which has a half life of 7.1×10^8 years and decays to ^{231}Th which, as before, is radioactive and decays with a half life of 24.6 hours to ^{231}Pa. After six alpha decays and three beta decays, the series terminates with stable ^{207}Pb. Each member of the series has a mass number which is divisible

TABLE 5-3. — THE URANIUM (4N + 2) SERIES; ONLY MAJOR
DECAY MODES ARE LISTED

RADIONUCLIDE	RADIATION	HALF-LIFE
^{238}U	alpha	4.5×10^{10} years
^{234}Th	beta	24.1 days
^{234}Pa	beta	1.14 minutes
^{234}U	alpha	2.35×10^5 years
^{230}Th	alpha	8.0×10^4 years
^{226}Ra	alpha	1.62×10^3 years
^{222}Rn	alpha	3.82 days
^{218}Po	alpha	3.05 minutes
^{214}Pb	beta	26.8 minutes
^{214}Bi	beta	19.7 minutes
^{214}Po	alpha	1.5×10^{-4} seconds
^{210}Pb	beta	22 years
^{210}Bi	beta	5.0 days
^{210}Po	alpha	138 days
^{206}Pb	none	stable

TABLE 5-4. — THE ACTINIUM (4N + 3) SERIES; ONLY THE PRINCIPAL
RADIONUCLIDES ARE LISTED

RADIONUCLIDE	RADIATION	HALF-LIFE
^{235}U	alpha	7.1×10^8 years
^{231}Th	beta	24.6 hours
^{231}Pa	alpha	3.2×10^4 years
^{227}Ac	beta	21.7 years
^{227}Th	alpha	18.9 days
^{223}Ra	alpha	11.2 days
^{219}Rn	alpha	3.92 seconds
^{215}Po	alpha	1.83×10^{-3} seconds
^{211}Pb	beta	3.61 minutes
^{211}Bi	beta	2.16 minutes
^{211}Po	alpha	5×10^{-3} seconds
^{207}Pb	none	stable

by four with a remainder of three, so the series is known as the 4n + 3 series. All of the members are given in Table 5-4. The reason why ^{235}U and other members of the series are rare relative to ^{238}U is the much shorter half life of ^{235}U relative to ^{238}U. More ^{235}U has decayed since the formation of the solar system.

The thorium (4n) series. — The thorium series begins with the long-lived thorium isotope ^{232}Th, which has a half life of 1.4×10^{10} years. After four beta decays and six alpha decays, the stable end product is ^{208}Pb. The complete series is given in Table 5-5; each radioisotope in the series has a mass number which is evenly divisible by four, so the series is also known as the 4n series.

Many of the members of the three series were discovered before the true nature of radioactive decay was understood, and they were designated as UX_1, Thorium A, Radium D, *etc.* After 1913, when the chemical

TABLE 5-5. — THE THORIUM (4N) SERIES

RADIONUCLIDE	RADIATION	HALF-LIFE
^{232}Th	alpha	1.4×10^{10} years
^{228}Ra	beta	6.7 years
^{228}Ac	beta	6.13 hours
^{228}Th	alpha	1.90 years
^{224}Ra	alpha	3.64 days
^{220}Rn	alpha	54.5 seconds
^{216}Po	alpha	0.16 second
^{212}Pb	beta	10.6 hour
^{212}Bi	beta	60.5 minutes
^{212}Po	alpha	3×10^{-7} seconds
^{208}Pb	none	stable

consequences of decay were proposed by Rutherford and Soddy, the chemical uniqueness of each of the members of the series was recognized.

There is a possible fourth series of radioactive isotopes, but this series (4n + 1) does not occur in nature, apparently because no member of the series has a half life long enough to have survived since the creation of the earth. The longest-lived member of the 4n + 1 series is ^{237}Np, which has a half life of only 2.2×10^6 (2.2 million) years.

Other naturally occurring radioisotopes. – In addition to the heavy elements making up the three radioactive series, several other elements have radioactive elements which occur in nature. The most interesting is ^{40}K, an isotope of potassium which has a half life of 1.3×10^9 years and makes up 0.012% of the naturally-occurring isotopes of potassium. ^{39}K (93.1%) and ^{41}K (6.9%) are stable. Since the human body contains about 150 Gm. of potassium, ^{40}K is one of the main sources of radiation to which a person is exposed during his lifetime.

Another naturally-occurring radioactive isotope is rubidium-87, which has a half life of 5×10^{10} years and decays to stable ^{87}Sr. This isotope is the basis for the rubidium-strontium dating technic for very ancient rocks and has been one of the main methods for establishing the age of lunar rocks.

Although ^{40}K and ^{87}Rb were apparently produced in the events which gave the earth its present elemental distribution, a radioactive isotope of carbon, ^{14}C, is being continually produced by cosmic ray bombardment of the nitrogen (^{14}N) in the earth's atmosphere. Carbon 14 has a half life of only 5,760 years and is incorporated into the carbon of all living things. When a tree, animal or person dies, ^{14}C is no longer accumulated, and the amount of ^{14}C decreases with the half life mentioned above. By measuring the ^{14}C content of any carbon-containing relic of the past, it is possible to determine when the sample was alive. The technic of carbon 14 dating is useful back to several thousand years B.C., but rests on the assumption that the rate of production of ^{14}C has been constant over that period.

The naturally-occurring radionuclides mentioned in this section are the principal sources of radiation exposure to the general population. In addition to the radiation from ^{40}K, there is also the exposure from natural sources of uranium and radium, which release radioactive radon gas into the atmosphere. The consequences of this exposure are discussed more fully in Chapter 9.

Artificial Radioactivity

The term artificial radioactivity refers to radioactive nuclei produced by man. More than 1,500 nuclei which are unstable with respect to decay have been produced since 1932, when the neutron was discovered. The number of artificial radioisotopes greatly exceeds the number of natural radionuclides, and only artificial radioisotopes are used in nuclear medicine.

Two basically different types of radioactive nuclei can be differentiated: those which have an excess of neutrons and those with a deficiency of neutrons. This broad division separates the radioactive isotopes into two groups, each of which has properties and methods of production which are fundamentally different.

Radioactive nuclei with an excess of neutrons.—With the advent of nuclear reactors, which are a prodigious source of neutrons, it has become possible to produce a large number of radioactive isotopes which have an excess of neutrons. Recall that a neutron has a mass of one atomic mass unit (A.M.U.) and carries no charge, so that a neutron may easily enter the nucleus and be captured by it. Thus, by simply inserting a sample of material into a nuclear reactor, neutrons are captured by the nuclei of the sample, thereby activating it.

A typical example of neutron capture is the production of ^{99}Mo in a reactor by irradiating naturally occurring molybdenum metal, which contains 23.78% of the stable isotope ^{98}Mo. The nuclear reaction is written in a shorthand form which is very similar to chemical reaction equations:

$$^{98}_{42}\text{Mo} + n = {}^{99}_{42}\text{Mo (radioactive)}. \tag{5-5}$$

In addition to the neutrons which are produced as a result of the fission of the uranium or plutonium fuel in a reactor, each fission of the fuel nuclei produces two lighter fragments, called fission products, which are usually radioactive. Many different elements, from gallium (atomic number 31) to lutetium (atomic number 71), are produced in the fission process which splits the uranium nucleus into two products of unequal size. One possible fission reaction might be written:

$$^{235}_{92}\text{U} + n \xrightarrow{\text{fission}} {}^{131}_{53}\text{I} + {}^{101}_{39}\text{Y} + 2n. \tag{5-6}$$

Both fission products have a large excess of neutrons, and both are radioactive. Among the isotopes used in nuclear medicine which are produced as fission products are ^{131}I and sometimes ^{99}Mo (which is the parent of ^{99m}Tc).

The decay properties of all neutron-excess nuclei are basically similar: they decay by emission of a beta (β) particle. The process of beta decay is discussed in detail below.

Radioactive nuclei with a deficiency of electrons.—Neutron-deficient nuclei have assumed a greater importance in nuclear medicine because of their unique decay properties, which are discussed later. The production of neutron-deficient nuclei costs energy—energy to remove one or more neutrons from the nucleus. This energy is usually supplied by bombarding the nucleus with a proton, deuteron, or alpha particle which has been accelerated in an atom-smashing device such as a cyclotron or linear accelerator. These machines are usually very large, requiring a building of their own, and they consume large amounts of power. Therefore, they are expensive to operate and, in addition, require a substantial capital investment. Most machines accelerate particles with electrostatic forces. The simplest machine of this type, a Van de Graaff accelerator, is sketched in Figure 5-3. In the Van de Graaff accelerator, positive charges are transferred by means of the moving belt from the high voltage power supply to the sphere (corona cap) at the top of the generator, where a large positive charge is built up. Positive ions (hydrogen-H, helium-^{4}He) are released inside the corona, and are repelled by the large positive charge. The Van de Graaff accelerator can operate continuously, with beam currents of the order of one microampere (6×10^{12} particles per second). This current can transform 6×10^{12} nuclei per second and produce fairly large quantities of activity—millicurie amounts or more, depending on the half-life of the radioisotope being produced (see following section).

The most popular machine for production of neutron-deficient radionuclides is the cyclotron, which is depicted schematically in Figure 5-4. The dees are evacuated chambers which are located between the poles of a large magnet. Charged particles are forced into a circular path by the

Fig. 5-3.— Simplified diagram of a Van de Graaff accelerator.

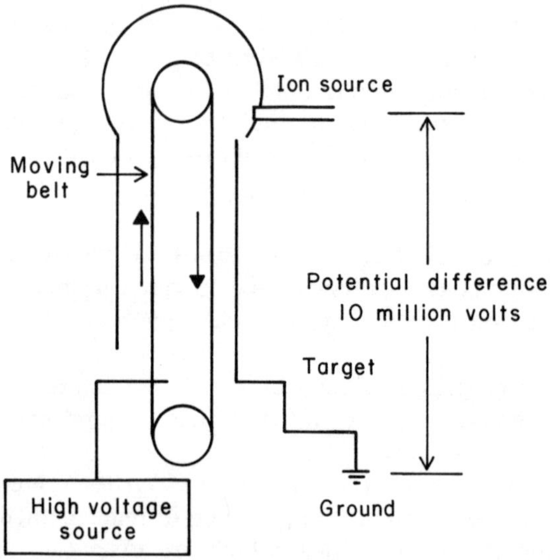

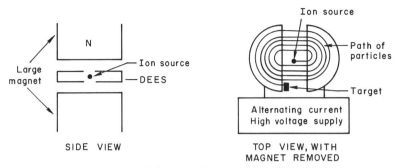

Fig. 5-4. — Schematic drawing of cyclotron.

magnetic field. Positive ions are released in the region between the two dees. An alternating high voltage is applied to the dees—the first one is positively charged, and the other is negative. The potential difference between the dees accelerates the particles, which are then forced into a circular path inside one of the dees. By the time the particle has reached the edge of the dee, after completing a half-circle, the sign of the charge on the dees has changed; the particle receives another boost and travels a semicircular path with a slightly larger radius in the second dee. The process continues until the particle reaches the target region, which may be inside or outside the dees. Cyclotrons may have beam currents of the order of several milliamperes, so the quantities of radioisotopes which can be produced may be curies or more, again depending on the half-life of the radionuclide involved.

One great advantage of accelerator-produced radioisotopes is that they are usually made in the carrier-free state. For example, ^{123}I is produced by the reaction ^{122}Te(p, γ)^{123}I. The ^{123}I product is the only iodine isotope present and it is thus carrier-free. Other radioisotopes of importance in nuclear medicine which are produced by charged-particle bombardments are ^{87}Y (parent in the ^{87}Y-^{87m}Sr generator) and ^{18}F. With the development of industrial and hospital-based cyclotrons, the number of accelerator-produced radionuclides used in nuclear medicine is certain to increase.

Equation for the production of radioisotopes. — Whether radioisotopes are produced by neutron irradiation or in a cyclotron, the basic equation for the production of radionuclides is the same:

$$A = C\left(1 - e^{\frac{-0.693\,t}{t_{1/2}}}\right) \tag{5-7}$$

in which A is the amount of activity, C is a constant which will be discussed in more detail below, t is the time of irradiation, and $t_{1/2}$ is the half-life of the radioisotope being produced. If the irradiation time is much shorter than the half-life, the equation can be reduced to:

$$A \text{ (millicuries)} = \frac{C \times 0.693 \times t}{t_{1/2}}. \qquad (5\text{-}8)$$

When a neutron-excess isotope is being produced in a reactor the constant C is given by

$$C = 1.6 \times 10^{-8} \frac{w\,\phi\,\sigma}{\text{At. Wt.}} \text{ (millicuries)} \qquad (5\text{-}9)$$

in which w is the sample weight in grams, ϕ is the neutron flux of the reactor in neutrons per second per square centimeter, σ is the cross-section for the nuclear reaction (a measure of how likely a neutron is to be captured by a nucleus) in barns, and At. Wt. is the atomic weight of the element being irradiated. The constant C is sometimes called the

Fig. 5-5.—Plot of the exponential part $(1 - e^{\frac{-0.693t}{t_{1/2}}})$ of equation 5-7, expressed as a percentage of saturation as a function of the number of half-lives the target is irradiated. The curve is valid for any radioisotope produced by any method.

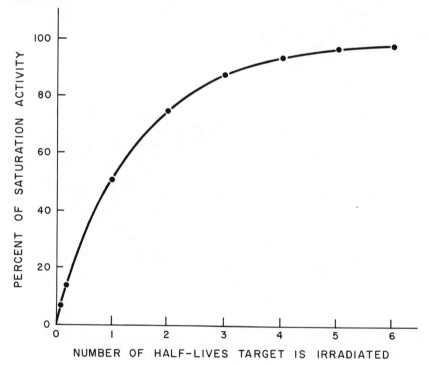

TABLE 5-6.— FACTORS TO BE CONSIDERED IN THE IRRADIATION OF
NATURAL MOLYBDENUM METAL FOR THE PRODUCTION OF ^{99}Mo

Nuclear reaction	^{98}Mo (n, γ) ^{99}Mo
Isotopic abundance of ^{98}Mo	23.78%
Amount of metal irradiated	100 grams
Neutron flux in reactor	10^{14} neutrons/cm.^{2}/sec.
Cross-section	0.5 barn
Time of irradiation	67 hours (one half life)

saturation term, since it is the maximum amount of radioactivity which can be produced. A limit is reached because some of the radioactive atoms are decaying; at saturation, the number being produced by neutron irradiation or charged-particle bombardment is exactly equal to the number decaying.

Returning to equation 5-7, the activity is seen to be the saturation term (C) multiplied by an exponential term which includes the half life of the isotope being produced. Figure 5-5 is a plot of the exponential term — the percentage of saturation reached as a function of the number of half lives the target is irradiated. The figure is valid for any radioisotope produced by any continuous method of irradiation — neutrons or charged particles. The interesting point in Figure 5-5 is that 50% of the saturation activity is obtained in one half life and it literally takes forever to make the remaining 50%. Thus, it is not economical to irradiate a sample for more than one half life.

As an example, let us consider the production of ^{99}Mo by the neutron irradiation of natural molybdenum metal. The pertinent data for this irradiation are given in Table 5-6. Since the irradiation is done for one half life, we expect to reach 50% of the saturation. The problem reduces to a calculation of the saturation term C. Substituting the values from Table 5-6 into equation 5-9, we have

$$C = \frac{(1.6 \times 10^{-8})(100 \times 0.2378)(10^{14})(0.5) \text{ millicuries}}{98}$$

(5-10)

$$= 1.94 \times 10^5 \text{ millicuries.}$$

The over-all yield, corrected for irradiation time, is then 9.7×10^4 millicuries. The factor 0.2378 is required because not all the atoms in molybdenum are the isotope ^{98}Mo.

Since many isotopes used in medicine are produced by fission of ^{235}U in a nuclear reactor, it is of interest to calculate the saturation term C for fission-produced radionuclides. For short-lived nuclei, the usual procedure is to irradiate a sample of ^{235}U and not wait for the reactor to be shut down for reloading. Consider the irradiation of ^{235}U for the production of ^{99}Mo in a reactor. In this case, the cross-section for fission (σ_f) of ^{235}U by neutrons is the term used for σ. Another important quantity is the fission yield (Y) of ^{99}Mo; that is, what fraction of the fission events produce ^{99}Mo. The equation for the saturation term C is now

$$C = \frac{(1.63 \times 10^{-8})(w)(\sigma_f)(\phi)(Y_{99_{Mo}})}{\text{At. Wt.}} \text{ millicuries.} \tag{5-11}$$

The fission cross-section of ^{235}U is 80 barns, and the fission yield of ^{99}Mo is 0.06 (6%). (The values of the fission yields are available in a number of reference sources.) Using the same reactor as described in Table 5-6 for one gram of ^{235}U, C is found to be 3.27×10^4 mCi. An important point in this method of producing ^{99}Mo for ^{99}Mo-^{99m}Tc generators is that the ^{99}Mo is carrier-free; in the irradiation of molybdenum metal, there is a considerable amount of stable molybdenum present. This means that generators made with fission-product ^{99}Mo require a much smaller amount of absorbent to hold the molybdenum on the generator. The point is discussed in greater detail in the following section.

Radioactive Decay Processes

There are a number of different radioactive decay processes, but only the three main types will be discussed in detail in this text. The three important and different types were discovered early in this century, and were named for the first three letters of the Greek alphabet: alpha (α), beta (β), and gamma (γ). As in the case of x-rays, the radiations were soon identified as helium nuclei (α), electrons (β), and high energy photons (γ); however, and again as with x-rays, the original names have been retained.

It should be recalled that all radioactive decay processes release energy from the nucleus and that the decays are spontaneous. The energy available for decay is simply the mass difference between the initial nucleus and the final nucleus plus any decay products. If the mass difference is in atomic mass units, the decay energy in MeV is given by:

$$E_{\text{decay}} \text{ (MeV)} = 931.7 \times \text{amu.} \tag{5-12}$$

Both natural and artificial radioisotopes decay by the three main processes. These are discussed below.

Alpha decay. — Alpha decay is the spontaneous emission of a helium nucleus by a (usually) heavy nucleus. A general equation for the alpha decay process can be written as

$$^{A}_{Z}X_N \rightarrow \,^{A-4}_{Z-2}Y_{N-2} + \,^{4}_{2}He_2. \tag{5-13}$$

Alpha decay has the following effects: the atomic number (Z) is reduced by two, creating a new element; the atomic weight (A) is decreased by four units and the number of neutrons (N) is reduced by two. All the alpha particles emitted by one alpha-emitting nuclide usually have the same energy, but there may be several groups of alpha particles with different energies. This is shown in the decay schemes of two alpha-emitting isotopes, ^{210}Po, and ^{238}U, which are illustrated in Figure 5-6, together with their spectra. Polonium 210 has only one alpha group with an energy of 5.305 MeV; ^{238}U has several groups which result from alpha decay from ^{238}U to various energy states in ^{234}Th. Thus, alpha decay involves a transition from the ground state of one nucleus (the "parent") to the ground state or excited levels in the product nucleus (the "daughter").

The spectra shown in Figure 5-6 are typical for naturally-occurring alpha decay nuclides which emit alpha particles with energies in the range of 4 to 8 MeV. The energy of the alpha group or groups is characteristic of the radioisotope, and learning the amount of energy present is an important step in the identification of an unknown alpha-emitting radioisotope.

The spectrum of any type of nuclear radiation is usually plotted as in Figure 5-6, i.e., the number of particles with a given energy as a function

Fig. 5-6.— Alpha decays of ^{210}Po and ^{238}U, illustrating the groups of alpha particle energies associated with each decay.

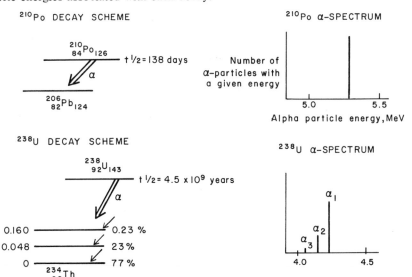

of energy. This type of graph is important, and it is worth the effort to understand what is being shown because this type of graph will appear again in connection with other decay processes.

Alpha-emitting isotopes are of very little interest in nuclear medicine, but ^{226}Ra is still used extensively in cancer radiotherapy. The process is discussed here because it is a relatively simple decay event and serves as a basis for development of more complex decay processes.

Beta decay. — The name beta (β) decay is applied to three different decay processes, all of which are similar in that they follow the same kind of physical laws and involve the spontaneous emission of electrons (or positrons, which are exactly like electrons except that they carry one positive charge) or the capture of electrons by the nucleus.

ELECTRON EMISSION. — The most familiar type of beta decay is electron emission. Inside the nucleus, a neutron is converted to a proton and an electron plus a neutrino are emitted, as follows:

$$_Z^A X_N \rightarrow \,_{Z+1}^A Y_{N-1} + e^- + \bar{\nu}. \tag{5-14}$$

The effect of electron emission is to increase the atomic number (Z) by one, creating a new element, and decrease the neutron number (N) by one. There is no change in atomic weight (A). The neutrino is a nearly weightless, neutral particle first postulated by Pauli in 1931 to account for the fact that all of the electrons emitted were not of the same energy, a fact which seemed to violate the law of conservation of energy. It was not until 1956 that the neutrino was observed and positively identified by Reines and Cowan in an experiment which allowed all physicists to breathe a bit easier.

Unlike alpha particles, which are emitted in mono-energetic groups, electrons (and positrons) emitted in beta decay have a range of energies from zero to the maximum energy difference between the parent and daughter nuclei. The decay scheme and beta particle spectrum of ^{32}P, a typical beta emitter, are shown in Figure 5-7. The decay scheme of ^{32}P is

Fig. 5-7. — The decay scheme and beta spectrum of ^{32}P. The electrons have a range of energies from 0 to 1.7 MeV, the energy difference between ^{32}P and ^{32}S.

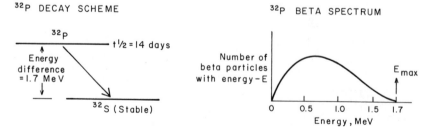

^{32}P DECAY SCHEME ^{32}P BETA SPECTRUM

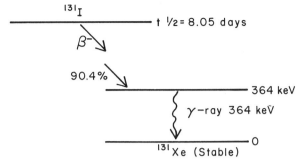

Fig. 5-8.—The simplified decay scheme of ^{131}I.

simple, with a transition energy from the ground state of ^{32}P to ^{32}S being 1.7 MeV, but not all the beta particles are emitted with an energy of 1.7 MeV, as would be expected from the discussion of alpha decay. In fact, the average beta particle energy is about one third of 1.7 MeV or 0.6 MeV. This approximation is valid for most beta emitters. The remainder of the decay energy goes to the neutrino, which is nearly weightless and has no charge, and is thus not usually detected.

It is also possible to have beta decay from the ground state of the parent to an excited state of the daughter nucleus. This is in fact what happens in the beta decay of ^{131}I, as shown in the simplified decay scheme of Figure 5-8. Here, some of the beta-decay transitions go to an excited state in ^{131}Xe, which de-excites by emitting a gamma ray of 364 keV, the gamma ray that is used to detect the beta decay of an atom of ^{131}I.

POSITRON EMISSION.—Positron emission occurs in nuclei which are neutron deficient. A proton is converted to a neutron inside the nucleus, and a positron and a neutrino are emitted. The general equation is

$$_Z^A X_N \rightarrow {}_{Z-1}^A Y_{N+1} + e^+ + \nu. \tag{5-15}$$

The effects of positron emission are: the atomic number (Z) is decreased by one, creating a new element; the neutron number (N) is increased by one; and the atomic weight (A) is unchanged. For positron emission to occur, the energy difference between parent and daughter nuclei must be at least 1.02 MeV. If this quantity of energy is not available, the nucleus will decay by electron capture, as discussed in the next section.

As in electron beta decay, the positrons emitted have a range of energies, from 0 to ($E_{max} - 1.02$ MeV), as shown in Figure 5-9, which depicts the decay scheme and positron spectrum of ^{18}F. Once again, the decay energy ($E_{max} - 1.02$ MeV $- E_{\beta^+}$) which does not go to the positron ends up with a neutrino. The ultimate fate of the positron is to interact with an electron in a dance of death called annihilation and to pro-

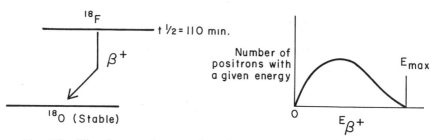

Fig. 5-9.—The decay scheme and positron spectrum of ¹⁸F. The maximum decay energy of ¹⁸F is 1.66 MeV, and the maximum positron energy is 0.54 MeV.

duce two gamma rays of 511 keV. The process of annihilation is discussed in greater detail in the next chapter.

ELECTRON CAPTURE.—Electron capture is a beta-decay process that is not accompanied by charged-particle emission. The nucleus in this case captures an atomic electron, and in the process a proton is converted to a neutron inside the nucleus. A neutrino is emitted in the decay event, which is given by the general equation

$$\,^A_Z X_N + e^- \rightarrow \,^A_{Z-1} Y_{N+1} + \nu. \tag{5-16}$$

The net effect of electron capture is the same as in positron decay: the atomic number (Z) is decreased by one, creating a new element; the neutron number (N) is increased by one; and the atomic weight (A) remains unchanged. In addition, the capture of an atomic electron by the nucleus creates a vacancy in the electron shells. When this vacancy is filled by an electron from a higher shell, an x-ray characteristic of the daughter nucleus is emitted. This process was discussed in detail in Chapter 2. The emission of characteristic x-radiation is the *only* easily observable phenomenon associated with electron capture. If enough decay energy is available to remove an electron from the innermost (K) shell of the parent nucleus, the process is called K-electron capture. Electron capture can also occur in the L, M, and higher shells.

As mentioned in the section on positron decay, electron capture is competitive with positron emission. Electron capture is the *only* decay mode available to neutron-deficient nuclei which are heavier than their daughter nuclei by less than 1.02 MeV. When the decay energy is more than 1.02 MeV, both positron emission and electron capture may occur. A typical case of electron capture is depicted in Figure 5-10, which shows the decay scheme of ⁵⁵Fe. The decay energy of ⁵⁵Fe is 231 keV, so the only mode of decay available is electron capture. The only observable external manifestation of the decay is an extremely weak K x-ray of Mn, with an energy of 6 keV.

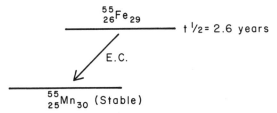

Fig. 5-10.—The decay scheme of ^{55}Fe.

Another case, in which electron capture and positron emission are competitive is ^{22}Na, as shown in the decay scheme of Figure 5-11. In ^{22}Na, 90% of the decays are by positron emission, and 10% occur through electron capture. The total decay energy is 2.841 MeV, enough for positron decay, and yet electron capture still occurs. The ^{22}Na decay scheme also indicates that most of the decay goes to the ^{22}Ne level at 1.275 MeV, which subsequently de-excites by emitting a gamma ray with this energy.

The importance and usefulness of the quantum-mechanical model of the atom is shown in the process of electron capture. The Bohr model (see Chapter 2) would have the electrons circling at some distance from the nucleus, and it is difficult to see how electron capture could occur under these circumstances unless the nucleus were much larger than indicated. However, using the quantum-mechanical model (see Fig. 2-5) in which it is necessary that the electron actually spend some of its time inside the nucleus, it is obvious how the electron can be captured by the nucleus.

The half lives of beta emitters vary from fractions of a second to many millions of years. The general rule for all three types of beta decay is the greater the decay energy, the shorter the half life, all other things being

Fig. 5-11.—The decay scheme of ^{22}Na.

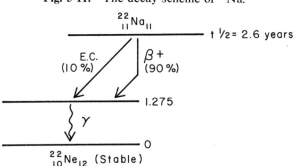

equal. Some of these "other things" are discussed in greater detail in the next sections.

Gamma decay.—Gamma (γ) rays are very short-wavelength, electromagnetic radiation emitted in the process of nuclear decay. The gamma ray is produced when the nucleus rearranges itself from one energy state to a lower energy state. There is no change in atomic weight (A), atomic number (Z), or the neutron number (N). The general equation is

$$_Z^{Am}X_N \rightarrow _Z^{A}X_N. \qquad (5\text{-}17)$$

Typical gamma-ray emitters are ^{99m}Tc and ^{113m}In. The process of gamma decay is of primary importance in nuclear medicine, since most procedures performed depend on the emission and detection of gamma rays. The process is so important and so central to understanding the physics of nuclear medicine that we devote the following separate sections to the phenomenon of gamma decay.

Gamma Rays and Nuclear Isomerism

The presence of the letter "m" in the superscript of the notation ^{99m}Tc indicates that the nucleus is metastable. Most metastable nuclei are in excited states and return to the ground state, releasing the excitation energy by gamma-ray emission. Excited nuclear states with half lives in the easily observable range of seconds to years are called isomers, and often carry the letter "m" in their superscripts, as ^{99m}Tc (6.0 hours), ^{113m}In (100 minutes), and ^{110m}Ag (250 days). In fact, isomers are known with half lives ranging from less than 10^{-12} seconds to 600 years. The theoretic reason for this spread in half lives for gamma-ray emission is based on quantum-mechanical models of the nucleus itself. As with the atom, models of nuclear structure have been proposed that explain (and help visualize) what is going on inside the nucleus. Although no one model provides a satisfactory explanation of all nuclear phenomena, the so-called shell model of the nucleus does well in explaining nuclear isomerism. In the shell model, nuclear properties are dominated by the quantum characteristics of one or two nucleons (a collective name for neutrons and protons). Thus all nuclei have a set of quantum numbers associated with their various energy states. The two important quantum numbers for nuclear decay are spin (I) and parity (Π). Not too inaccurately, nuclear spin can be thought of as how fast the nucleus is spinning. The nuclear spin is quantized; that is, it may have only certain integer (0, 1, 2, *etc.*) or half-integer (1/2, 3/2, 5/2, *etc.*) values. Nuclei with an even number of protons and an even number of neutrons (even-even nuclei) have integral spins, with the ground state being zero. Odd-even

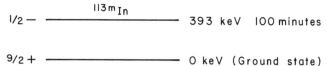

Fig. 5-12.—The level scheme for the isomers of ¹¹³In. The first excited state has a spin-parity assignment of 1/2 –; the ground state spin is 9/2 and the parity is even (+).

and even-odd nuclei have half-integral spins, and odd-odd nuclei have integral spin values.

The concept of parity is more difficult to explain without recourse to quantum mechanics. Briefly, the solution of a nuclear wave equation produces a three-dimensional mathematical representation of the nucleus. If the representation is symmetric with respect to inversion through the center of symmetry, the parity is said to be even (+); otherwise, the parity is odd (–). A spheric shape would have + parity, but a cone would have – parity. Commonly, nuclear spin parity assignments are written beside a line representing the nuclear energy level, as shown in Figure 5-12 for ¹¹³ᵐIn.

The spin and parity are quantities which can be determined in rather complex experiments.

The lifetimes of nuclear isomeric states depend mainly on the changes in spin and parity. All other things being equal, the greater the spin change (ΔI), the longer the lifetime, and a decay requiring change in parity ($\Delta \Pi$) takes longer than a decay in which no change is required. In addition, the more energetic the gamma-ray decay is, the faster it goes. These rules, which are also valid for alpha and beta decay, are summarized in Table 5-7. We now apply these rules to the decay of ⁹⁹ᵐTc, for which the decay scheme is shown in Figure 5-13.

On the basis of the information provided, γ_1 and γ_2 lifetimes are ex-

TABLE 5-7.—THE EFFECTS OF SPIN, PARITY AND ENERGY
CHANGE THE HALF-LIFE FOR ALPHA-, BETA-, AND
GAMMA-RAY DECAY
(In each tabular entry, the other changes
are assumed to be negligible.)

QUANTITY CHANGED	CHANGE	EFFECT ON HALF-LIFE
Parity ($\Delta \Pi$)	No	Decreased
Parity ($\Delta \Pi$)	Yes	Increased
Decay energy (ΔE)	Increased	Decreased
Decay energy (ΔE)	Decreased	Increased
Spin (ΔI)	Increased	Greatly increased
Spin (ΔI)	Decreased	Greatly decreased

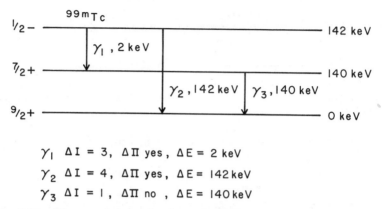

γ_1 $\Delta I = 3$, $\Delta \Pi$ yes, $\Delta E = 2$ keV

γ_2 $\Delta I = 4$, $\Delta \Pi$ yes, $\Delta E = 142$ keV

γ_3 $\Delta I = 1$, $\Delta \Pi$ no , $\Delta E = 140$ keV

Fig. 5-13.—The complete level scheme for ^{99m}Tc. The spin, parity and energy changes for all gamma-ray transitions are also given.

pected to be slow, with γ_1 being faster than γ_2 because the smaller spin change ($\Delta I = 3$ *vs.* $\Delta I = 4$ for γ_2) overwhelms the larger energy change ($\Delta E = 2$ keV *vs.* $\Delta E = 142$ keV for γ_2). The γ_3 transition is exceptionally fast, with a half life below 10^{-9} seconds.

The gamma rays emitted by ^{113m}In and in the decay of ^{131}I are rather close—393 and 364 keV, respectively—so that it is of interest to look at the effect of spin and parity changes in these cases. The decay schemes are given in Figure 5-14.

Notice that the 364 keV gamma ray usually attributed to ^{131}I actually is the disintegration of a nuclear level in ^{131}Xe. The prolongation of the ^{113m}In lifetime by 15 orders of magnitude results mainly from the large spin change ($\Delta I = 4$).

Fig. 5-14.—The decay scheme of ^{113m}In and the partial decay scheme of ^{131}I. The lifetimes are different by 15 orders of magnitude.

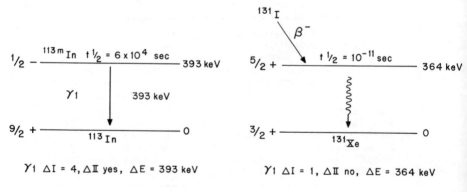

The process of nuclear decay by emitting a gamma ray is not the only way in which an excited nuclear level can get rid of its excess energy and reach the ground state. An alternative to gamma-ray emission is internal conversion in which the decay energy is given to one of the atom's atomic electrons. This process is discussed in the next section.

Gamma Rays and Internal Conversion

The process of internal conversion is the de-excitation of a nucleus by an interaction with the atomic electrons. In internal conversion, an excited nucleus decays to the ground state not by emitting a gamma ray, but by giving up its energy to an atomic electron. The longer the lifetime of an isomeric state, the more likely it is that internal conversion will take place. This is another case in which the wave-mechanical model of atomic structure (see Chap. 2) provides helpful information. In the Bohr model, it is difficult to conceive of how the nucleus can interact with the atomic electrons, but with the quantum-mechanical model the interaction is credible, since the electron is believed to spend some part of its time in the nucleus where it can easily acquire the excitation energy of the nucleus. A comparison of ^{113m}In and ^{131}I is again instructive in illustrating the effects of lifetime on internal conversion. For ^{113m}In, about 35% of the transitions from 393 keV to the ground state go via internal conversion. Internal conversion is only 2% for ^{131}I. The electron through which the nuclear level de-excites is emitted by the nucleus with an energy equal to the decay energy minus the binding energy of the electrons in the shell from which they are removed. Internal conversion may take place in any atomic shell, as in the case of electron capture. The amount of internal conversion associated with a gamma-ray transition is designated by the quantity α_K, α_L, α_M, *etc.*, which indicate the ratio of K-, L-, and M-shell conversion electrons emitted to gamma rays emitted. This information is usually included in the information given with the decay scheme. All the information known about the decay of ^{99m}Tc is given in Figure 5-15. Note that the 140 keV transition is about 10% internally converted in the K-shell ($\alpha_K = 0.1$). Thus, of 100 transitions from the 140 keV level in ^{99m}Tc, 90 result in a 140-keV gamma ray, and 10 K-shell conversion electrons, each with an energy of 119 keV (140 keV − 21 keV, the K-shell binding energy for Tc) are emitted.

The internal conversion process is very important since it produces energetic electrons; these high-energy electrons can contribute a significant portion of the internal radiation dose from an injected isotope. It is often falsely stated that ^{99m}Tc emits *only* gamma rays and is thus a "safer" isotope. However, as we have just seen, there are also conversion elec-

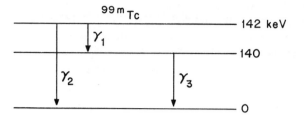

$$\gamma_1 : \ 2\ keV \quad \alpha \gg 1$$

$$\gamma_2 : \ 142\ keV \quad \alpha_K = 0.10, \ K/L = 8.1$$

$$\gamma_3 : \ 140\ keV \quad \alpha_K = 29, \ K/L = 3.2$$

Fig. 5-15.—The level scheme for ^{99m}Tc, including all known information on internal conversion of gamma-ray transitions in the decay of ^{99m}Tc. The fraction K/L is the ratio of internal conversions in the K-shell to that in the L-shells.

trons to be considered. This problem is considered in greater detail in Chapter 7.

Since internal conversion creates a vacancy in one of the atom's electron shells, there is emission of characteristic x-rays when the vacancy is filled by electron transitions from higher shells. This is another way in which internal conversion is similar to the process of electron-capture decay. The internal conversion process resulting in the emission of characteristic x-rays is responsible for the only external radiation (K-characteristic x-rays) observable in the decay of ^{125}I. The decay scheme of ^{125}I is shown in Figure 5-16. Decay from the 0.035 keV level in ^{125}Te to the ground state is almost completely by the internal conversion process. This results in tellurium K-characteristic x-rays with energies of approximately 28 keV. These x-rays are in addition to those produced in the electron-capture decay itself.

Fig. 5-16.—The decay scheme of ^{125}I.

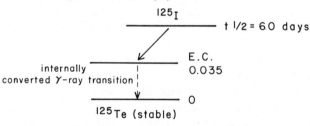

Radionuclide Generators

The decay of a radionuclide usually produces a stable product. However, a large number of radioactive nuclei decay to daughter nuclei which are themselves radioactive. The three naturally-occurring radioactive series mentioned at the beginning of this chapter are examples of this multiple decay process. A number of pairs of radioactive nuclei have been developed specifically for the production of radioisotopes for nuclear medicine. The parent-daughter relationship is exploited to produce a generator, or cow. Usually the parent has a longer half life than the daughter, although this is not an absolute requirement for a generator system.

The basic equations giving the amount of daughter activity in a parent-daughter system were solved some years ago by Bateman and the equations bear his name. For any parent-daughter system, the general solution to the Bateman equation is

$$A_2 = \frac{\lambda_2}{\lambda_2 - \lambda_1} A_1^0 (e^{-\lambda_1 t} - e^{-\lambda_2 t}) + A_2^0 e^{-\lambda_2 t} \qquad (5\text{-}18)$$

in which A_2 is the daughter activity at any time t,
$\quad \lambda_1$ is the decay constant of the parent,
$\quad \lambda_2$ is the decay constant of the daughter
$\quad A_1^0$ is the initial activity of the parent, and
$\quad A_2^0$ is the initial activity of the daughter.

Equation 5-18 can be applied to any parent-daughter system, but there are two special cases which are of particular interest to nuclear medicine. The first case is when the parent has a longer half life than the daughter; in equation 5-18, $\lambda_2 > \lambda_1$. This situation produces the state known as transient equilibrium. This means that after sufficient time has elapsed there will be a constant ratio between the numbers of parent and daughter atoms. This can be seen by examining equation 5-18 for large values of time: the $e^{-\lambda_2 t}$ and $A_2^0 e^{-\lambda_2 t}$ terms become very small. Then

$$A_2 = \frac{\lambda_2}{\lambda_2 - \lambda_2} A_1^0 e^{-\lambda_1 t} \qquad (5\text{-}19)$$

and since $A_1 = A_1^0 e^{-\lambda_1 t}$, the ratio of activities is given by

$$\frac{A_1}{A_2} = \frac{\lambda_2 - \lambda_1}{\lambda_2}. \qquad (5\text{-}20)$$

Here it can be seen that the ratio of activities of parent and daughter can vary between 0 and 1, depending on the size of λ_1 and λ_2.

We now return to equation 5-18 and ask what is the time course of activity of the daughter in a parent from which the daughter atoms have just been separated. That is, the "cow" has just been "milked." The case of the ^{99}Mo-^{99m}Tc generator system will be considered in detail. Here $\lambda_1 = 0.693/67 = 0.01033$ hour^{-1}, and $\lambda_2 = 0.693/6.0 = 0.1155$ hour^{-1}. In the case just mentioned, ^{99m}Tc has just been removed, so the second term, A_2^0, is zero.

First, consider the parent, ^{99}Mo; it continues to decay with a half-life of 67 hours, so the activity decreases with this half life, as shown in Figure 5-17. Using the exponential values in Appendix C, it is a simple matter to solve equation 5-18 for values of A_2 as a function of time. These values are given in Table 5-8, together with the number of millicuries of ^{99m}Tc produced in the generator. The ^{99m}Tc data are also plotted in Figure 5-17, where it can be seen that the ^{99m}Tc content grows to about one half of the ^{99}Mo content in 6.0 hours, or one ^{99m}Tc half life. Notice that as time goes on the amount of ^{99m}Tc in the generator is a function of the ^{99}Mo half life only, since the $e^{-\lambda_2 t}$ term becomes very small (< 0.001) after 60 hours. It should also be noted that there is actually more ^{99m}Tc than ^{99}Mo in the generator after about 23 hours.

Fig. 5-17. – A case of transient equilibrium. Growth of ^{99m}Tc in a ^{99}Mo – ^{99m}Tc generator; note that the activity scale is logarithmic.

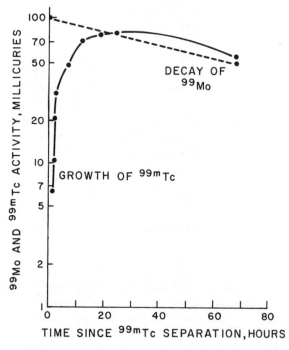

TABLE 5-8.—SOLUTION OF EQUATION 5-18 FOR THE ^{99}Mo$-^{99m}$Tc
GENERATOR SYSTEM*

TIME FROM MILKING IN HOURS	$e^{-\lambda_1 t}$	$e^{-\lambda_2 t}$	$e^{-\lambda_1 t}-e^{-\lambda_2 t}$	A_2, mCi ^{99m}Tc
0.5	1.000	0.942	0.058	6.4
1.0	0.990	0.896	0.094	10.3
2.0	0.980	0.795	0.185	20.3
3.0	0.970	0.705	0.265	29.0
6.0	0.942	0.500	0.442	48.5
12.0	0.887	0.250	0.637	70.0
18.0	0.827	0.125	0.702	77.0
24.0	0.779	0.062	0.717	78.6
48.0	0.613	0.031	0.582	64.0
67.0	0.500	0.000	0.500	54.9
72.0	0.477	0.000	0.477	52.3
96.0	0.333	0.000	0.333	36.6
134.0	0.250	0.000	0.250	27.4

*These data show the growth of ^{99m}Tc in a generator which initially contained 100 mCi of ^{99}Mo and has just been "milked" of ^{99m}Tc. This means that A_1^0 = 100 mCi, and A_2^0 is zero. From data given in test, $\lambda_2/\lambda_2 - \lambda_1 = 1.097$.

The second case of equation 5-18 which is of particular interest to nuclear medicine is when the half life of the parent is much longer than that of the daughter. This is the case with the ^{113}Sn-^{113m}In generator system, in which ^{113}Sn has a half life of 115 days, whereas ^{113m}In has a half life of 1.75 hours. For time periods of less than a few days, the decay of ^{113}Sn can be neglected ($e^{-\lambda_1 t} = e^0 = 1.00$), and λ_1 is negligible

TABLE 5-9.—SOLUTION OF EQUATION 5-21, AN EXAMPLE OF
SECULAR EQUILIBRIUM*

TIME FROM MILKING IN HOURS	$(1 - e^{-\lambda_2 t})$	A_2, mCi ^{113m}In
0.01	0.004	0.04
0.02	0.007	0.07
0.05	0.020	0.20
0.10	0.039	0.39
0.20	0.076	0.76
0.50	0.181	1.81
1.0	0.330	3.30
1.75	0.500	5.00
2.0	0.546	5.46
3.50	0.750	7.50
5.00	0.861	8.61
5.25	0.875	8.75
10.0	0.981	9.81
24.0	0.999	10.0

*These data show the growth of ^{113m}In in a ^{113}Sn − ^{113m}In generator after complete removal of ^{113m}In.

relative to λ_2 ($\lambda_1 = 0.00025$ hour^{-1}, $\lambda_2 = 0.396$ hour^{-1}), so equation 5-18 reduces to

$$A_2 = A_1^0 (1 - e^{-\lambda_2 t}).\qquad(5\text{-}21)$$

Equation 5-21 gives the growth of ^{113m}In in a ^{113}Sn-^{113m}In generator which has just been milked. The values for the exponential part of the equation and A_2 are given in Table 5-9 for a generator which contains 10.0 mCi of ^{113}Sn. The data are also plotted in Figure 5-18, in which it can be seen that the ^{113m}In activity increases to 50% of the ^{113}Sn activity in 1.75 hour, the ^{113m}In half life, then to 75% in two half lives. Ultimately, the activities of both ^{113}Sn and ^{113m}In are equal; this is then called secular equilibrium. The Bateman equations for a long chain of radioactive decay products—such as the three naturally-occurring chains mentioned earlier—show that in an undisturbed sample of uranium or thorium, all the members of the decay chain are in secular equilibrium. That is, all the radionuclides have exactly the same disintegration rate.

Other Modes of Decay

Although of very limited usefulness in nuclear medicine at the present time, several other decay processes should be mentioned to complete

Fig. 5-18.—A case of secular equilibrium. Growth of ^{113m}In in a ^{113}Sn–^{113m}In generator. The activity scale is logarithmic.

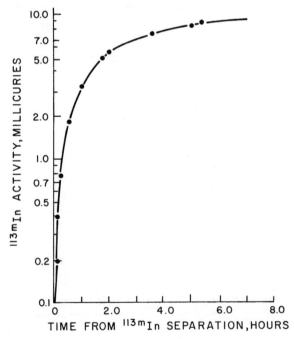

TIME FROM ^{113m}In SEPARATION, HOURS

the list. The process of spontaneous fission (S.F.) is interesting and may become an important source of neutrons. Certain very heavy natural and artificial radionuclides spontaneously decay by fission. For example, ^{235}U and ^{238}U can undergo fission, which competes with alpha decay. A heavy man-made isotope of Californium, ^{252}Cf, undergoes S.F. in about 3% of its decays. Recall that the fission of any heavy nucleus usually produces several neutrons, and it can be seen easily that a few grams of ^{252}Cf can be a source of an enormous number of neutrons (2.3×10^{12} neutrons/sec./Gm.). Research is now being directed toward using these neutrons to produce radiographs in much the same way that x-rays are used to produce diagnostic radiographs.

Two rather esoteric forms of radioactive decay are neutron and proton emission. Both of these processes require that the nucleus acquire a large amount of energy, usually more than 5 MeV. Instead of going through a gamma-ray transition, the excited nucleus kicks out one of its nucleons to reach a lower energy configuration.

We have now presented a complete discussion of radioactivity, including all types and kinds. The next step in the learning process will be to understand how this radiation interacts with matter and how it is detected and measured. These complex subjects are taken up in the next chapter, but rely heavily on the knowledge obtained here.

SUGGESTED READING

Blahd, W. H. (ed.): *Nuclear Medicine* (2d ed.; New York: McGraw-Hill Book Company, Inc., 1971), Chap.1.
Friedlander, G., Kennedy, J. W., and Miller, J. M.: *Nuclear and Radiochemistry* (2d ed. New York: John Wiley and Sons, Inc., 1964), Chap. 2.
Glasstone, S.: *Sourcebook on Atomic Energy* (New York: D. Van Nostrand Co., Inc., 1950), Chap. 5.
Johns, H. E.: *The Physics of Radiology* (2d ed.; Springfield, Ill.: Charles C Thomas, Publisher, 1964), Chap. 3.
Selman, J.: *The Fundamentals of X-Ray and Radium Physics* (4th ed.; Springfield, Ill.: Charles C Thomas, Publisher, 1965), Chaps. 21, 22.

STUDY QUESTIONS

1. Define the half life of a radioisotope.
2. Using the table of exponentials (Appendix C), determine the amount of ^{131}I remaining in a sample which contained 15.0 mCi initially at 2, 5, 15, 20 and 80 days.
3. Calculate the decay constants of the following radionuclides: ^{18}F, ^{99m}Tc, ^{131}I, and ^{203}Hg. Express all decay constants in the same units.
4. A sample of ^{99m}Tc originally contained 10.0 mCi. Calculate the disintegration rate (counts per minute) at 1.0, 4.0 and 8.0 hours.
5. Provide at least two definitions of specific activity.
6. Define carrier-free radioactive material.

7. A sample of ^{125}I contains 5.0 mCi of ^{131}I in the carrier-free state. What does the iodine in the sample weigh?

8. Give three examples of naturally-occurring radioactive materials that are *not* members of the three naturally-occurring decay chains.

9. Explain why the examples chosen in problem 8 are still present on the earth.

10. Give two different methods for producing artificial radioactivity.

11. Write a general equation for alpha decay.

12. The alpha decay of ^{210}Po produces an alpha particle with an energy of 5.30 MeV. How much mass is converted to energy in the decay of ^{210}Po? Answer in amu and grams.

13. What is the major feature of electron and positron emission as compared to alpha decay?

14. Explain why the neutrino is required in beta decay.

15. Write general equations for the three types of beta decay.

16. Compare electron capture with positron emission.

17. Explain electron capture in terms of the quantum-mechanical model of the nucleus.

18. What are the two alternative ways of de-excitation of a nuclear energy level above the ground state.

19. Give the effects of spin, parity and energy on the half life of a nuclear isomer.

20. A ^{99m}Tc generator initially contained 300 mCi of ^{99}Mo and has not yet been milked. Three days after the calibration date, how much ^{99m}Tc will be available from the generator, assuming 100% yield?

21. The generator mentioned in problem 20 is milked again four hours later. How much ^{99m}Tc will be produced?

22. How long will it take for the generator of problem 20 to decay to 10 μCi of ^{99}Mo?

CHAPTER 6

Detection and Measurement of Nuclear Radiation

THE DETECTION AND MEASUREMENT OF NUCLEAR RADIATION is a fundamental step in nuclear medicine. The radiation emitted by radioactive materials in the patient or test sample is counted with nuclear medicine equipment. However, the interactions of radiation with matter must be understood before the actual detection of radiation can be mastered, for these interactions are the basis for the design of detection systems.

Types of Nuclear Radiations

Nuclear radiations of interest in nuclear medicine consist of alpha, beta, and gamma radiations. Alpha particles are energetic helium ions emitted by the nucleus. Beta particles are electrons or positrons emitted in nuclear decay processes. Gamma rays are high-energy, short-wavelength, electromagnetic radiation emitted by a nuclear isomer which may have a half life of less than 10^{-12} second to over 100 years.

Interaction of Radiation with Matter

PARTICULATE RADIATION

Since nuclear radiation can be divided into two classes, particulate (alpha and beta) radiation and electromagnetic (gamma ray) radiation, the two classes will be discussed separately. One of the early observations made about alpha and beta rays was that these particles are absorbed fairly easily. Alpha particles may be absorbed completely by a sheet of paper. Consider the experiment shown in Figure 6-1, which is set up to avoid the inverse-square dependence law.

If the source-to-detector distance is increased, the count rate will remain almost constant and then drop sharply, as shown in the figure. The distance denoted Rα is known as the range of the alpha particle, and is related to the alpha particle energy, as follows:

$$R = 0.318 \, E^{+3/2} \qquad (6\text{-}1)$$

55

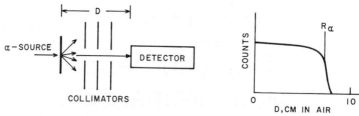

Fig. 6-1.— An experiment designed to determine the range (*R*) of alpha particles in air. Collimators are used between the source and detector to provide a beam of alpha particles of constant count rate.

in which R is the range in centimeters and E is the alpha-particle energy in MeV. The alpha particles lose energy as they pass through matter, chiefly by ionization of matter. Ionization is a process of removing electrons from atoms, creating free electrons (e⁻) and positive ions. Using a cloud chamber, it is possible to measure the amount of ionization along the track of an alpha particle. The result of such a measurement is shown schematically in Figure 6-2. The amount of ionization is fairly constant initially, then rises to a maximum, then falls abruptly. The shape of the curve is dependent on the energy of the alpha particle, which decreases as the path increases since it costs some energy to ionize an atom or molecule of absorber material. As the alpha particle loses energy, more ionization is possible. Toward the end of the range, the helium ion (He⁺⁺) may pick up an electron to become He⁺, which is less ionizing. This process is called straggling, and accounts for small differences in the ranges of individual alpha particles.

Alpha-particle ranges are usually measured in air under standard conditions (+15 C., 760 mm. Hg pressure). In air, as in most gases, the energy lost by ionization amounts to about 35 ev per ion pair. The relationship between energy and range may be seen more clearly in terms of

Fig. 6-2.— The rate of ionization along the track of an alpha particle.

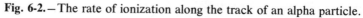

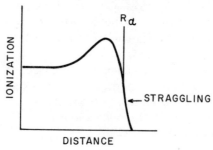

the energy loss per unit path length—often called LET (linear energy transfer) or dE/dX. For 5 MeV alpha particles in air, the LET varies along the path, as shown in the previous diagram, but ranges from 70 to 210 keV/mm. It should be noted that the LET includes the energy imparted to the electrons after ionization. A theoretic equation has been derived to express LET as a function of the physical properties of the incident particle and the absorber:

$$LET = A \frac{z^2 N Z}{v^2} \log \frac{(Bv^2)}{I} \qquad (6-2)$$

in which A and B are constants, z is the charge of the incident particle, N is the number of atoms per cubic centimeter of the absorber of atomic number Z, v is the speed of the incident particle, and I is the average excitation potential of the absorber. The important points in the equation are the linear dependence of LET on N and Z and the square dependences for z and v.

Beta particles (electrons and positrons) are much more penetrating than alpha particles, as indicated in Table 6-1. Since beta ranges in air are so large, solid absorbers are often used instead of gases. Usually beta ranges are quoted in terms of the superficial density of absorber, because beta ranges are then nearly independent of absorber material. The superficial density is simply the thickness of the absorber multiplied by its density. The units of superficial density are thus grams or milligrams per square centimeter. If an experiment similar to that described for alpha particles is performed with a beta emitter and aluminum absorbers, the results would be as shown in Figure 6-3. The result is, fortuitously, a straight line on a semilog plot, and the count rate as a function of absorber thickness is given by

$$C = C_o e^{-\mu x} \qquad (6-3)$$

in which C is the count rate after passing an absorber of thickness X, μ is the absorption coefficient, and C_0 is the count rate with no absorber in place. The passage of beta particles through matter is more complex than the passage of alpha particles. For example, the electron may lose most of its energy in a single collision, so straggling may be great. Also, since the electron is so light, scattering by atomic electrons in the absorb-

TABLE 6-1.—THE RANGES AND LET VALUES FOR 3MEV
ALPHA AND BETA PARTICLES IN AIR

PARTICLE	ENERGY	RANGE IN AIR	LET
$\alpha(\text{He}^{++})$	3 MeV	2.8 cm.	100,000 ev/mm.
$\beta(\text{e}^-$ or $\text{e}^+)$	3 MeV	1,200.0 cm.	150 ev/mm.

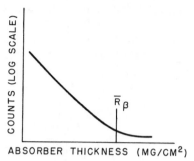

Fig. 6-3.—Results of an experiment designed to determine the range of beta particles (either e^+ or e^-) in an absorber.

er may be large. In addition to energy loss by ionization, another process called bremsstrahlung can become an important source of energy loss for high-energy beta particles. Bremsstrahlung (literally, slowing down radiation) is emitted when an electron is decelerated in the electric field of the nucleus. The relative amounts of energy lost by the two processes are computed as follows:

$$\frac{(LET) \text{ Bremsstrahlung}}{(LET) \text{ Ionization}} = \frac{EZ}{800} \tag{6-4}$$

in which E is the beta particle energy in MeV, and Z is the atomic number of the absorber. Incidentally, the bremsstrahlung process is responsible for the production of x-rays in an x-ray tube. Accelerated electrons are slowed down in a tungsten target (Z = 74). For 100-keV electrons, the bremsstrahlung process converts about 1% of the electron energy into x-rays; the remainder of the electron beam energy is ultimately converted to heat.

An additional interesting phenomenon occurs when the beta emission happens to be positrons. The passage of positrons through matter produces exactly the same effects as electrons, i.e., ionization and bremsstrahlung. However, when the positron comes to rest it combines with an electron in a process called annihilation. The two particles cease to exist and their mass is converted into two 511-keV gamma rays which are emitted in opposite directions. The process of annihilation occurs whenever matter (such as electrons) meets antimatter (such as positrons). Since the positron-electron annihilation takes place when the positron has come to rest, the momentum of the positron-electron system is close to zero. The two 511-keV gamma rays are emitted in opposite directions in order to conserve momentum (one of the basic conservation laws of physics). The annihilation process is depicted in Figure 6-4. Notice that

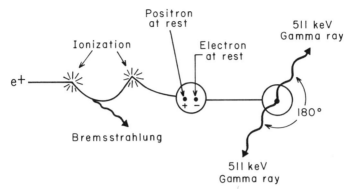

Fig. 6-4.—The annihilation process. When the positron comes to rest after giving up all its energy by ionization and bremsstrahlung, it interacts with an electron in a process called annihilation. The positron and electron disappear, and their mass appears as two 511-keV gamma rays emitted at 180 degrees to each other.

after annihilation both positron and electron cease to exist. The 511-keV gamma rays produced in annihilation are characteristic of all positron emitters; the 511-keV gamma ray is known as annihilation radiation.

Electromagnetic Radiation

The passage of x- or gamma rays through matter also produces ionization; however, scattering plays a much more important role in the interaction of high energy photons than is the case with alpha or beta particles.

The LET for photons is one tenth to one hundredth that of an electron of the same energy. There are four distinct mechanisms by which gamma and x-rays interact with matter. Each of the four processes tends to predominate in a particular energy region.

CLASSICAL SCATTERING

In this interaction, which is also known as coherent scattering, only the direction of an incident photon changes; there is no loss of energy. The process is analogous to changing the direction of a light beam with a mirror. This mechanism is important only at very low energies—below one keV.

PHOTOELECTRIC ABSORPTION

In photoelectric absorption, the total energy of the photon is transferred, in a single event, to an atomic electron, which is then knocked out of the atom. The gamma ray must have at least enough energy to dis-

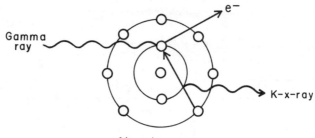

Absorber atom

Fig. 6-5.—The photoelectric absorption process. The gamma ray gives all of its energy in a single collision to an atomic electron. The electron goes on to give up its energy by ionization and bremsstrahlung in the absorber. A characteristic x-ray is also produced.

Fig. 6-6.—Relative probability of various photon interactions for three absorbers, for photons of energy from 100 keV to 10 MeV. For very light elements (low atomic number), the Compton process predominates over the entire energy region.

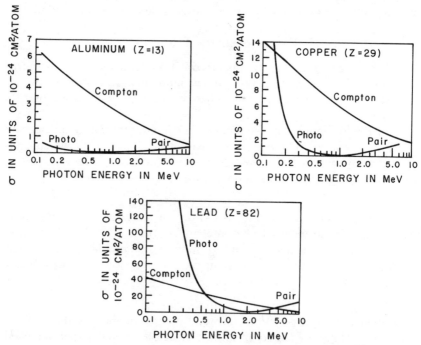

lodge the atomic electron from its particular shell. For example, the binding energy of the K-shell electrons in iodine is 33 keV. A 50-keV gamma ray could interact with a K-shell atomic electron in iodine, knock it out of the shell, and also provide the free electron with 17 keV of kinetic energy. The energetic electron would then interact with the absorber, just like a beta particle, as described earlier. Since the iodine atom now has a vacancy in the K-shell, there is a rearrangement of the atomic electrons which produces characteristic x-rays. These x-ray photons will interact further with the absorber, usually by a photoelectric interaction with a higher shell electron. The photoelectric absorption process is depicted in Figure 6-5. In a good scintillation crystal such as sodium iodide, the complete process described above takes less than 10^{-9} second. The photoelectric effect tends to predominate at energies between 1 keV and 500 keV in heavy elements, although the photoelectric cross-section is quite dependent on the atomic number of the absorber, as shown in Figure 6-6.

COMPTON SCATTERING

The Compton effect can be viewed as an elastic (billiard ball) collision between the incident photon and a free electron. (Strictly speaking, no electrons in an absorber are free or unbound to a nucleus. However, the binding energy of an outermost electron in any atom is only a few electron volts [ev], which is negligible when compared to a gamma ray of several hundred keV.) The incident photon transfers some of its energy to the electron, which then can interact with the absorber by ionization and bremsstrahlung as mentioned earlier. Since the incident photon loses some energy to the electron, the wavelength of the photon is increased. The scattered gamma ray may go on to interact with the absorber by further Compton events, or may give up all its energy in a photoelectric process. It is also possible that the scattering angle may be such as to allow the scattered gamma ray to leave the absorber. In the latter case, only a portion of the incident gamma-ray energy will be absorbed in the form of the recoil electron. The Compton process is sketched in Figure 6-7. Compton scattering of the gamma ray may occur with any angle (ϕ) up to 180 degrees (backwards). The energy lost to the recoil electron may be determined by:

$$E_{recoil} = E\gamma \left[\frac{\alpha(1 - cos\ \phi)}{1 + \alpha(1 - cos\ \phi)} \right]$$

(6-6)

in which Eγ is the gamma-ray energy in MeV, α is equal to Eγ in MeV divided by 0.511, and ϕ is the scattering angle of the scattered photon. If the photon hits the free electron straight on, the electron goes straight

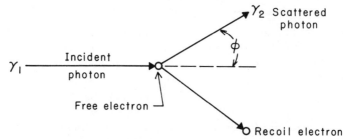

Fig. 6-7.—The Compton effect. Only part of the incident photon's energy is given up to the free electron. The recoiling electron goes on to interact with the absorber by ionization and bremsstrahlung. The Compton-scattered gamma ray may interact further with the absorber by any of the four processes described in the text.

ahead and the scattered gamma ray goes back in the direction whence it came ($\phi = 180$ degrees). This gives the electron the most energy, since cos 180 degrees $= -1$. Substituting this value in equation 6-6 gives the maximum electron recoil energy

$$E_{\text{recoil}_{(\text{max.})}} = E\gamma\left(\frac{2\alpha}{1 + 2\alpha}\right). \tag{6-7}$$

For low-energy photons, most of the energy is transferred to the recoil electron. Compton scattering tends to be the predominant interaction process over a wide range of gamma energies, especially for low-Z absorbers, as shown in Figure 6-6. However, all of the energy of a gamma ray may be given up to an absorber in a series of Compton events followed by a final photoelectric event, as shown in Figure 6-8.

Fig. 6-8.—Absorption of a gamma ray in an absorber by multiple Compton scattering, followed by a final photoelectric interaction. The whole process occurs in less than 10^{-9} second.

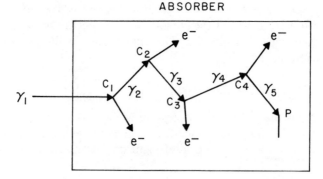

ABSORBER

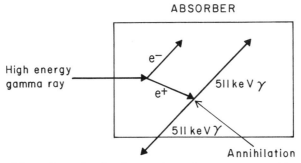

Annihilation

Fig. 6-9.—The pair-production interaction of gamma rays with matter. The high-energy gamma ray produces an electron-positron pair, giving up its energy in excess of 1.02 MeV to the particles, which go on to be absorbed as electrons. The final fate of the positron is to undergo annihilation, thereby producing two 511-keV gamma rays.

PAIR PRODUCTION

The pair-production interaction with matter requires a gamma ray with an energy of at least 1.02 MeV. As such, the process is not observed often in nuclear medicine, but it is very important in radiotherapy with high-voltage (greater than about 4 MV) machines. The high-energy gamma ray enters the absorber and, somewhere quite close to a nucleus, loses its identity and energy in the creation of an energetic electron-positron pair. The creation of this pair of particles requires 1.02 MeV of energy and is an example of the conversion of energy to mass. The energy equivalent of an electron or positron is 0.511 MeV, thus, to

TABLE 6-2.—THE INTERACTIONS OF GAMMA RADIATION WITH MATTER

INTERACTION	EFFECT ON GAMMA RAY	ENERGY RANGE IN WHICH INTERACTION IS IMPORTANT	SECONDARY EFFECTS
Classical scattering	No loss of energy; direction is changed	Below 1 keV	None
Photoelectric absorption	Total energy given up to atomic electrons, gamma rays disappear	Below about 500 keV	Energetic electrons, X-rays
Compton scattering effect	Some energy given up to "free" electrons	500 keV several MeV	Energetic electrons, scattered gamma rays
Pair-production interaction	Total energy given up to create $p^+ - e^-$ pair; gamma ray disappears	Above 5 MeV	Energetic electrons and positrons; annihilation radiation

create the electron-positron pair uses 1.02 MeV. If the gamma ray has more energy than 1.02 MeV, the excess energy is transferred to the electron and positron in equal amounts. The process is depicted in Figure 6-9. The electron and positron go on to interact with the absorber, as previously described. When the positron finally comes to rest, it undergoes annihilation, producing two 511-keV gamma rays. As indicated in Figure 6-6, pair production is a relatively unimportant mode of interaction of gamma rays for low atomic weight absorbers. The interactions of gamma rays with matter are summarized in Table 6-2 with the secondary effects given for each type of interaction.

The three main interaction processes are often summed to give a total absorption coefficient (μ) for gamma rays passing through matter. A

Fig. 6-10. – The half-thickness values of gamma rays in various absorbers. The half-thickness is quoted in milligrams per square centimeter (surface density). To obtain the half-thickness in centimeters, divide the value in milligrams per square centimeter by the density of the element in milligrams per cubic centimeter.

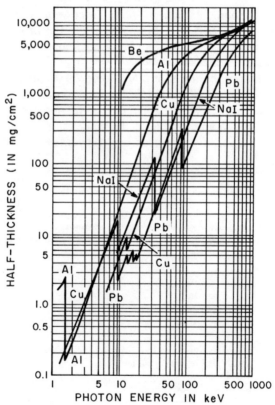

more convenient measure of the absorption is given by the thickness of absorber required to reduce a gamma-ray beam intensity to one-half its initial value. Here again, the thicknesses are given in terms of milligrams per square centimeter – the density multiplied by the absorber thickness. Half-thickness values for a number of absorbers are given in Figure 6-10.

Detection Systems

Perhaps the most striking characteristic of all the interactions of radiation with matter is the phenomenon of ionization – the production of free electrons and positive ions. Most useful detection systems (with the exception of scintillation counters) use this phenomenon to detect radiation.

IONIZATION COUNTERS

As the name implies, ionization chambers measure the ionization produced by the passage of radiation. Two oppositely-charged plates are set up, usually in air. According to the rules of electrostatics (defined in Chap. 4), the electrons created by the passage of ionizing radiation are attracted to a positively-charged plate, whereas the positive ions go to the negative plate. If there is a continuous source of ionization, there will be a continuous flow of electrons to the plates through an external circuit, as shown in Figure 6-11. Since current (amperes [AMPS]) is the rate of flow of electrons, the reading on the ammeter will be proportional to the ionization between the plates.

The current in the external circuit is quite small: 1.6×10^{-19} amps times the number of ion pairs per second. An important aspect of the operation of ionization chambers is the voltage on the plates. It must be high enough to draw all the ion pairs apart (to prevent recombination), yet not so high as to accelerate the electrons to the point at which fur-

Fig. 6-11. – A simple air ionization chamber. The region between the plates is the sensitive region of the detection system. Electrons (e⁻) are attracted to the positive plate, and positive ions (+) go to the negative plate.

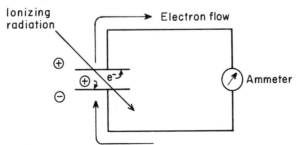

ther ionization occurs. A typical current-voltage curve for an ionization chamber is shown in Figure 6-12. When the plate voltage is low, the ions recombine to form neutral atoms before reaching the plate, so little current is observed. In the multiplication region, the electrostatic forces pulling the electrons to the positive plate supply enough energy to the electrons so that they become ionizing—i.e., capable of creating electron-positive ion pairs. The instrument should be operated at voltages in the "flat" region of the curve. For measurement purposes, the chamber must be calibrated with a source which is the same as, or quite similar to, the source being measured. The activity of the standard and unknown are then related to the amount of current produced by each source:

$$\frac{\text{Activity standard}}{\text{Current standard}} = \frac{\text{Activity unknown}}{\text{Current unknown}}. \qquad (6\text{-}8)$$

Ionization chambers are often used in nuclear medicine since they are very reliable and can be adapted easily to measure amounts of radioactivity between a few microcuries and many curies. Most current models have a built-in resistor or variable resistance circuit, so that the current reading on the ammeter reads directly in millicuries or microcuries of the radioisotope being measured. Some manufacturers have modified the instrument to provide a digital presentation of the activity so that the operator does not even have to read a dial.

Fig. 6-12.—The current-voltage curve for a typical ionization chamber. The instrument should be operated at voltages in the "flat" region of the curve.

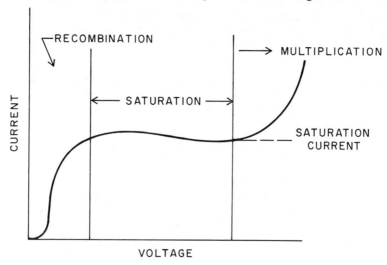

When using an ionization chamber of any type, care must be taken to standardize the instrument with a source of radioactive material which is identical, or nearly identical, with the radioisotope which is being measured. This requirement includes the type of radiation emitted by the material, the chemical and physical form of the isotope *and* the container material. Several manufacturers of radionuclides provide long-lived standards in multidose vials which simulate the properties of ^{99m}Tc and ^{131}I, as well as other radionuclides often used in nuclear medicine.

Portable ionization chambers, which obtained the somewhat strange name of "Cutie Pie" during the days of the Manhattan Project of World War II, are available and may be used for survey purposes. Such instruments are calibrated to read in milliroentgens or roentgens per hour and are invaluable in monitoring areas which may be contaminated by spilled radioactive materials and for measuring the radiation exposure in areas where radionuclides are produced and stored.

GEIGER COUNTERS

If the electrodes in an ionization counter are rearranged to form a central positively charged wire and a cylinder, the result is a Geiger-Müller (G-M) detector. In contrast to the ionization chamber, the G-M detector is usually operated to detect individual ionizing events. The current from each ionizing event is fed to a resistor-capacitor system which sets the time constant of the system, as shown in Figure 6-13.

The pulse of electrons charges up the capacitor, but the charge leaks off through the resistor. The time constant τ is defined as the time required for the capacitor charge to be reduced to $1/e$ ($= 0.368$) of its initial value, and its numerically given by $\tau = RC$, in which R is the resistance in ohms and C is the capacitance in farads. The operation of the G-M counter is most easily described by showing the size of the pulse output as a function of the applied voltage (see graph in Fig. 6-14). At low voltages, there is some recombination of ion pairs before they can be collect-

Fig. 6-13. — The basic circuit of a Geiger-Müller counter. Electrons are attracted to the center wire, which is positively charged.

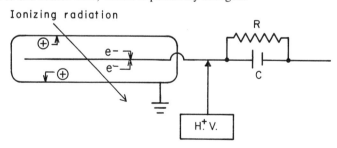

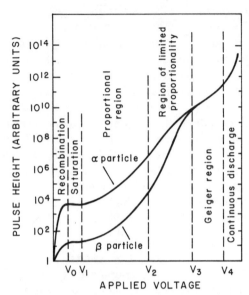

Fig. 6-14. – Variation of pulse height with applied voltage in a Geiger-Müller counter.

ed (up to V_0). In the region V_1 to V_2, the pulse height is proportional to the amount of energy deposited in the detector. There is some multiplication of ion pairs caused by acceleration of electrons. Above V_3, up to V_4, the creation of just one ion pair by ionizing radiation produces an avalanche of electrons on the center wire. This is the Geiger region in which all ionizing radiation, whether alpha, beta, or gamma, looks the same to the detector, and the G-M tube is usually operated in this region.

Portable Geiger counters are often used in nuclear medicine for survey work, i.e., to detect the extent and degree of contamination from a spill of radioactive material. Often these instruments are operated with four to six flashlight-type dry-cell batteries. They are simple and rugged, and an effective tool for monitoring alpha, beta and gamma radiation. Usually the instruments are calibrated to read in counts per minute and/or milliroentgens per hour.

One application of G-M detectors to diagnostic tests is their use in detecting certain tumors in the eye. Radioactive phosphorus (^{32}P) injected intravenously tends to accumulate in the tumor in 24 to 48 hours. Since ^{32}P is a beta emitter, the radiation must be detected by a detector placed directly on the eye. An eye probe, which is actually a G-M detector, is used to count the short-range beta particles.

METHODS NOT BASED ON ION COLLECTION

With the exception of scintillation counting, these methods are not of great importance in nuclear medicine, and are mentioned here simply for completeness. Photographic film is blackened by most types of electromagnetic radiation, and this property is employed to obtain (no-screen) x-ray and autoradiographic pictures. (Dental x-ray film is usually used in film badges for personnel monitoring.) Cloud chambers are used to detect ionizing radiation by maintaining a supersaturated vapor in an enclosed chamber. The ions apparently act as nucleation sites for condensation of the vapor. The bubble chamber, invented by Donald Glaser in 1952, makes use of the fact that liquids can be held at or above their boiling points for short periods of time without actually boiling. Bubble tracks are produced, apparently by local heating, along the path traversed by ionizing radiation through liquified gases, usually liquid hydrogen.

SCINTILLATION COUNTING

A number of organic and inorganic materials produce visible light when exposed to ionizing radiation, many for hours or days after excitation. There is considerable art – and not much science – in the production of light by ionizing radiation (TV picture tubes are a good example). Discussion here will be limited to the solid inorganic scintillator sodium iodide (NaI). By itself, pure NaI is not a good scintillator, but when between 0.1 and 0.5% thallium iodide is added, the light output increases more than tenfold; this is the commercial scintillator NaI(Tl). The material is grown as a single crystal from a melt. Since NaI(Tl) is hygroscopic (absorbs moisture from the air), it must be fabricated and used in an airtight system. A typical crystal-photomultiplier system is shown in Figure 6-15.

Remember that all the processes described for gamma radiation occur in the crystal. Some gamma rays produce photoelectrons, some undergo Compton scattering, and those with enough energy go through pair production. The light output of the scintillator is proportional to the energy deposited in the crystal. The light output of the scintillator is "looked at" by a photomultiplier tube (PMT). The visible light photons produced in the scintillator are conducted through a light pipe (usually lucite) to the PMT photocathode, where a number of electrons are knocked off by a photoelectric process. The photoelectrons are accelerated to the first dynode, where additional electrons are knocked out. This acceleration and multiplication process continues down the tube, until the last dynode is reached. The total multiplication (gain) in the phototube is a function of the high voltage on the photomultiplier tube: the higher the

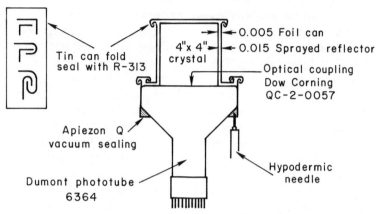

Fig. 6-15.—A scintillation crystal coupled to a photomultiplier tube (PMT) as an integral unit.

voltage, the larger the output pulse from the PMT. At this point, the voltage pulse produced by the photoelectric interaction of a gamma ray in the NaI(Tl) crystal followed by scintillation and photomultiplication may amount to a few millivolts. The process is shown schematically in Figure 6-16.

Two important aspects of the process must be stressed. First, the size of the output voltage pulse (the pulse height) is directly proportional to the amount of energy deposited in the NaI(Tl) crystal. Second, the emission of photoelectrons at the photocathode and the electron multiplication down the tube are statistical processes and so contribute some spread to the pulse height.

Fig. 6-16.—The conversion of gamma-ray energy to a voltage pulse using a scintillator crystal and photomultiplier tube.

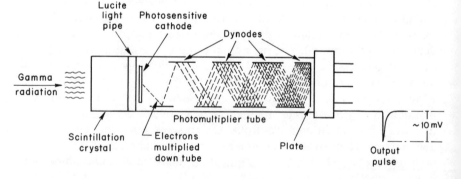

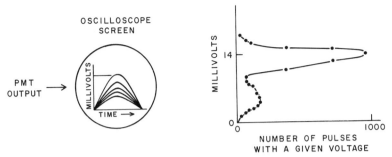

Fig. 6-17.—The output pulses of a PMT-NaI crystal exposed to the 140-keV gamma rays of ^{99m}Tc.

PULSE-HEIGHT ANALYSIS

To illustrate these effects, the output pulses of a photomultiplier tube-sodium iodide crystal which is exposed to the 140-keV gamma rays of ^{99m}Tc can be observed directly with an oscilloscope, as shown in Figure 6-17. The oscilloscope is an instrument designed to show voltage variations as a function of time, so many pulses appear to start at the same

Fig. 6-18.—Gamma-ray spectra of some isotopes used in nuclear medicine. The spectrum provides a method of identification in addition to the half-life.

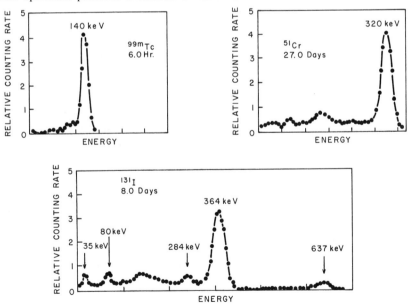

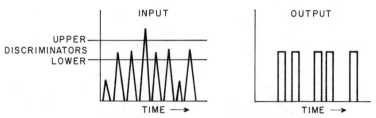

Fig. 6-19.—The operation of a simple pulse-height analyzer, with an upper and lower discriminator. Only those pulses meeting both upper and lower discriminator requirements produce an output pulse.

time. For the sake of convenience, we may adjust the high voltage to produce a pulse of about 14 millivolts (mv) when the 140-keV gamma ray undergoes a photoelectric interaction in the NaI crystal. Compton events in which the scattered gamma ray leaves the crystal produce smaller pulses. We observe a large number of pulses and then analyze the pulses by sorting them according to their height. We count the number of pulses with voltages between 0 and 1 mv, between 1 and 2 mv, *etc.*, as shown in the right side of Figure 6-17. The process just described is called pulse-height analysis (PHA) and is used in many nuclear medicine instruments. Pulse-height analysis produces a spectrum which is usually presented in the form shown in Figure 6-18. Again, we have the important graph of the number of counts of a given pulse height plotted as a function of the pulse height.

The width of the pulse heights selected is often called a window and may be large enough to include the whole photopeak of the gamma ray. The upper and lower edges of the window are called discrimination levels—the lower discriminator rejects pulses below the window and the upper discriminator rejects pulses above the window. By setting an upper and lower discriminator, it is possible to count only the photopeak of an isotope. In this way, ^{131}I can be distinguished from ^{99m}Tc. When an event does occur which meets the discriminator requirements, a uniform pulse is produced by the pulse-height analyzer. This pulse may be recorded on a counting scaler, sent to a rate meter system, or used in the recording of a scan. The process is illustrated schematically in Figure 6-19.

SEMICONDUCTOR DETECTORS

In the past 10 years, a new type of radiation detector has been intensively developed which has produced a small revolution in nuclear physics. The semiconductor radiation detector can be described as a solid-state ionization chamber. However, solids (the semimetals silicon or germanium) are about 1,000 times as dense as the gases used in ion chambers. In addition, the amount of energy required to produce an ion pair in silicon or germanium is only about 3 ev, or approximately one tenth of that needed for gases. Thus, electric signals are larger, statistic fluctuations smaller, and energy resolution significantly better, as shown in Figure 6-20.

The great improvement in energy resolution is apparent in the figure. This allows the clean separation and detection of a number of isotope pairs which cannot be easily resolved with NaI(Tl): for example, ^{131}I (364 keV) − ^{113m}In (393 keV), and ^{57}Co (122 keV) − ^{99m}Tc (140 keV).

Basically, a semiconductor is a material whose resistivity to the passage of electric current is about 10,000 ohm-cm. Good conductors have resistivities of the order of one ohm-cm., and good resistors (glass, plastics) have resistivities at 10^7 ohm-cm. or higher.

The major advantage of semiconductor detectors is their greatly increased energy resolution. There are several disadvantages of present materials which may preclude their rapid introduction into nuclear medicine. (1) The large lithium-drifted detectors Ge(Li) require constant refrigeration at liquid nitrogen temperatures (−320 F.). (2) The output of the detectors is only a few microvolts, so elaborate electronic amplifiers are required if full advantage of the improved resolution is to be realized. (3) Both silicon and germanium are less efficient than NaI(Tl) for gamma ray detection, mostly because of their lower atomic numbers. Develop-

Fig. 6-20. − The gamma-ray spectra produced by NaI(Tl) compared with a lithium-drifted germanium Ge(Li) detector.

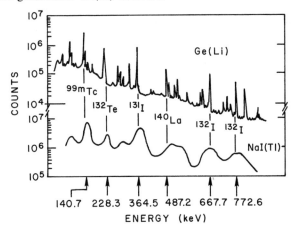

74   *Nuclear Medicine for Technicians*

ment of high-atomic-number semiconductor materials (bismuth telluride, for example) has been promised for several years; however, no commercial devices have appeared.

SUGGESTED READING

Blahd, W. H. (ed.): *Nuclear Medicine* (2d ed.; New York: McGraw-Hill Book Company, Inc., 1971), Chap. 1.
Friedlander, G., Kennedy, J. W., and Miller, J. M.: *Nuclear and Radiochemistry* (2d ed.; New York: John Wiley and Sons, Inc., 1964), Chap. 4.
Johns, H. E.: *The Physics of Radiology* (2d ed.; Springfield, Ill.: Charles C Thomas, Publisher, 1964), Chaps. 5, 6.
Quimby, E. H., Feitelberg, S., and Gross, W.: *Radioactive Nuclides in Medicine and Biology: Basic Physics and Instrumentation* (3d ed.; Philadelphia: Lea and Febiger, 1970), Chap. 7.
Selman, J.: *The Fundamentals of X-Ray and Radium Physics* (4th ed.; Springfield, Ill.: Charles C Thomas, Publisher, 1965), Chap. 12.

STUDY QUESTIONS

1. What is the principal difference between the interactions of alpha and beta particles with matter?
2. What are the main processes responsible for energy loss of alpha-particles in matter?
3. The average range of beta particles of ^{32}P is 2.00 mm. in water. What is the average range of these beta particles, expressed in milligrams per square centimeter?
4. What are the main processes responsible for energy loss of beta particles in matter?
5. Calculate the relative amounts of bremsstrahlung produced by a source of ^{32}P ($E_{\beta max} = 1.7$ mev) in absorbers of lead and copper. What can be said regarding the shielding of beta emitters to reduce the bremsstrahlung?
6. Describe the annihilation process for positrons.
7. What are the main processes responsible for energy losses of gamma rays in matter?
8. What phenomenon is common to all the interactions of all types of radiation with matter?
9. Describe how an ionization chamber operates.
10. What is the principal difference between the operation of an ionization chamber and a Geiger-Muller counter tube?
11. Describe the scintillation detection process from the interaction of gamma rays with the scintillator to the production of a voltage pulse at the last dynode of the photomultiplier tube.
12. Discuss the necessity for pulse-height analysis in the detection of gamma rays.

CHAPTER 7

Nuclear Medicine Instrumentation

THE INSTRUMENTATION OF NUCLEAR MEDICINE consists of gamma-ray cameras, rectilinear scanners, fixed detectors for counting in vitro samples, thyroid scintillation counters, and survey instruments. These instruments all have a number of features in common, and these parts will be discussed first to provide an overview of the machinery of nuclear medicine.

Common Features of Instrumentation

The basic detection system used in all nuclear medicine equipment is shown schematically in Figure 7-1. The system consists of a nuclear radiation detector surrounded by shielding to avoid the detection of extraneous radiation and fronted by a collimator so that only radiation arriving from a predetermined direction is detected. The detector is provided with high voltage from a power supply, and the detector output is coupled to an amplifier to increase the size of the output voltage pulses from the detector. The amplifier output is directed to a pulse-height analyzer to discriminate against unwanted events, and the pulse-height analyzer output is fed to some sort of display system. Several parts of the systems have been described elsewhere in this book—power supplies in Chapter 4, and detectors and pulse-height analyzers in Chapter 6.

A complete description of amplifiers is beyond the scope of this book; suffice it to say that amplifiers simply increase the size of the detector

Fig. 7-1.—Basic features of nuclear medicine instruments.

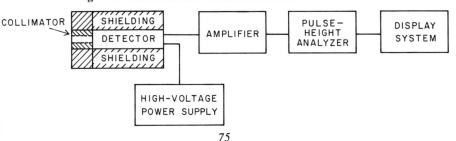

output pulse (e.g., from a pulse size on the order of a few millivolts, to one a few volts in size). The latter size is much easier for pulse-height analyzers to handle. The amplifiers are now completely transistorized, as is most of the equipment used in nuclear medicine, but there are still many hard-worked tube-type instruments in use.

The shielding around a detector usually is constructed of lead, which is a compromise between shielding and cost. A number of other materials (e.g., gold and tungsten) would make better shields, but their cost is prohibitive. Most sodium iodide scintillation detectors are surrounded by about one inch of lead. Figure 6-10 shows that this is sufficient shielding to absorb all but the highest energy gamma rays almost completely. The shielding surrounds the detector on three sides; the fourth side is left open for the detection of gamma rays which are emitted by the patient or sample under study. When used for in vitro studies, samples are placed on top of the scintillation crystal or in a well in the crystal and the fourth side of the detector is covered with shielding, again so that only the counts from the sample are detected.

The remaining parts of instrumentation systems in nuclear medicine — detectors, collimators and display systems — are important enough so that separate sections are devoted to them.

Detectors and Collimators

The detector in most nuclear medicine equipment is a sodium iodide scintillation crystal coupled to a photomultiplier tube. The crystal is usually in the form of a right circular cylinder, although detectors for in vitro counting often contain wells to increase the counting efficiency. Two typical NaI detectors are shown in Figure 7-2. The five-inch crystal, which is 2 inches thick, is typical of the crystal sizes used in present-day scanners, although many older instruments have only a three-inch diameter crystal. (Scanners derive their names from the diameter of the detector crystal).

In Chapter 6, it was mentioned that sodium iodide is hygroscopic; this is, NaI tends to absorb moisture from the air. Thus, the crystal must be completely covered to avoid destroying the scintillator. The crystals are usually "canned" in thin (0.010 inch) aluminum; for special applications, an entrance window of very thin (0.001 inch) aluminum or beryllium may be used. Such thin windows would be desirable if very low-energy gamma rays were to be counted. Often, the scintillation crystal, light pipe, and photomultiplier tube are canned as a single integral unit.

The light pipe is usually a disk of Lucite plastic that provides optical coupling between the NaI and the photomultiplier tube. The light pipe is

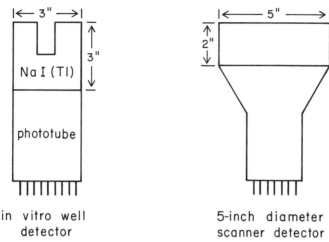

in vitro well
detector

5-inch diameter
scanner detector

Fig. 7-2.—Typical scintillation crystal-photomultiplier tube detectors used in nuclear medicine.

usually coated with silicone grease at the interface between the light pipe and the photomultiplier tube. The purpose of a light pipe is to provide an unobstructed path for the scintillator light from the NaI crystal to the phototube. The grease greatly decreases the reflection losses of light at the interface between the plastic light pipe and the glass envelope of the phototube. In gamma-ray cameras, which employ very large crystals and many phototubes, the light pipe may be cut so as to direct the light from one section of the crystal to one phototube in the array.

The NaI scintillation crystals in gamma-ray cameras are much larger in diameter (11 inches) and much thinner (1/2 inch) than the crystals in most scanners. The diameter of the crystal in the gamma-ray camera allows fairly large areas to be viewed by the camera, but the relative thinness of the crystal makes the camera very inefficient for high-energy gamma rays. The relative efficiency for a 1/2-inch thick NaI crystal for gamma rays of various energies is shown in Figure 7-3. The principal reasons for using a NaI crystal of only 1/2 inch in thickness are the scattering of scintillation light in the crystal and the increased likelihood of multiple Compton-scattering events (which could add up to the equivalent of a single photoelectric event) with thicker crystals. Most gamma-ray cameras employ a geometric arrangement of 19 phototubes which observe the scintillations in the NaI crystal through a light pipe. A typical arrangement of detector, light pipe, and photomultiplier tubes is shown in Figure 7-4.

The collimators used in nuclear medicine are usually constructed of

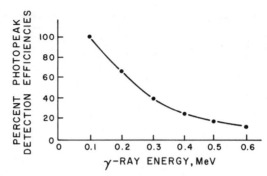

Fig. 7-3. — Relative gamma-ray photopeak detection efficiencies of a ½-inch thick NaI crystal.

lead metal. Collimators are designed to allow radiation to enter the detector from only one small region and to prevent radiation from other areas from being detected. The simplest collimator, which is often used for thyroid counting, consists of a single cylindric hole in a lead shield. A typical thyroid collimator and its field of view are shown in Figure 7-5. Note that there are two distinct regions below the collimator, the umbra, the area for which the collimator is most sensitive, and the penumbra, which defines the region of detectability below the collimator. Radiation emitted from regions outside the penumbra is not detected by the collimated crystal. The ratio of the area of the umbra to the area of the penumbra is decreased by tapering the collimator hole, as shown in Figure 7-6. In fact, at the focal plane of the collimator in Figure 7-6, the umbra is only a point. The cylindric, straight-hole collimator is the best system for thyroid counting.

All scanners use focused multihole collimators with tapered holes. These collimators are usually constructed of lead metal, which is easily cast by pouring the molten metal into a mold. The design of a good collimator is an art which requires the trading off of a number of factors,

Fig. 7-4. — A typical arrangement of detector, light pipe, and photomultiplier tubes in a gamma-ray camera.

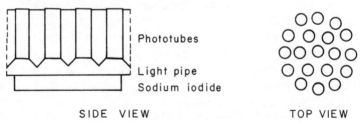

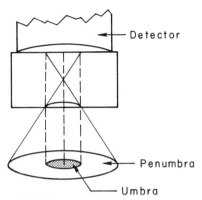

Fig. 7-5.—A single-hole collimator and its field of view. Such collimators are often used in thyroid-uptake studies. The umbra is the region in which the collimator is most sensitive. No radiation emanating from outside the penumbra region is detected.

such as efficiency and resolution. A simplified drawing of a multihole focused collimator is shown in Figure 7-7. The distance at which the fields of view of the individual holes superimpose is the focal distance. Collimators are named for their focal distance (3-inch, 5-inch, *etc.*). It can be seen how the focal distance might be varied by changing the angle of inclination of the holes.

The efficiency of a collimator is a measure of the number of counts permitted to reach the detector relative to the number of counts which would reach the detector in the absence of the collimator. A collimator with large tapered holes will be more efficient than one with smaller

Fig. 7-6.—A tapered-hole collimator. The ratio of the area of the umbra to the area of the penumbra is much smaller than in the straight-hole collimator.

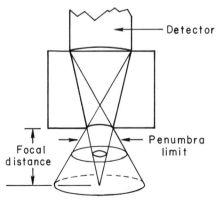

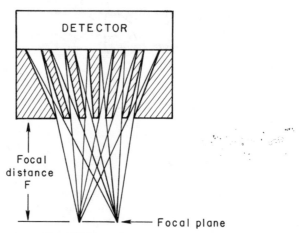

Fig. 7-7.—A simple multihole focused collimator. The fields of view of the individual holes superimpose only in the focal plane.

holes (since there is more lead in the latter), but the smaller-hole collimator will probably have finer resolution. The resolution is a measure of how well the collimator can distinguish a small amount of activity in an extended source containing a large amount of activity (as in a liver scan). The efficiency and resolution of a collimator are involved in a trade-off.

Fig. 7-8.— Response curve of a 3-inch fine collimator. The collimator cuts off more sharply in horizontal directions than in vertical directions.

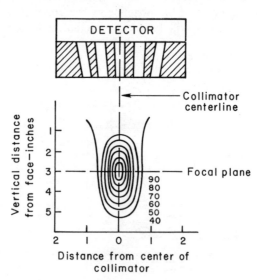

Increased resolution is obtained at the expense of decreased efficiency, and increased efficiency is purchased at the cost of decreasing resolution.

The response of a collimator is a measure of the efficiency of detection of radiation in the region in front of the detector, in both horizontal and vertical directions. The response curve of the typical collimator used in scanners has a much sharper cutoff in the horizontal direction than in the vertical area, as shown in Figure 7-8. This means that the collimator looks deeper (above and below its plane of focus), but that very little radiation is detected off the center line of the collimator.

Collimators for gamma-ray cameras are different from those of scan-

Fig. 7-9. — Collimators for gamma-ray cameras.

A. Straight hole, low energy

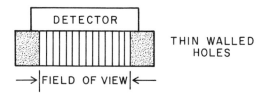

B. Diverging collimator, medium energy

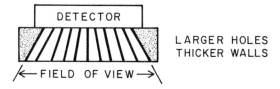

C. Pin hole collimator

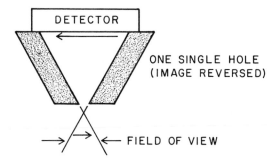

ners in that they are not focusing collimators. In fact, one collimator available with most cameras has holes which are diverging. The gamma-ray camera collimators are usually designed for optimum resolution and efficiency at a particular gamma-ray energy. Once again, these objectives are conflicting, and sacrifices in efficiency are made to improve resolution. More lead absorber is added between holes in high-energy collimators to prevent penetrating gamma rays from entering the crystal from the wrong direction. Typical collimators for a gamma-ray camera are shown in cross-section in Figure 7-9. The diverging collimator allows objects larger than the crystal to be imaged, and the pinhole collimator can provide magnification of small objects (for example, the thyroid gland). Low-energy collimators should never be used with isotopes which emit high-energy gamma rays; there will be considerable penetration of the lead shielding with a resulting blurred image.

Display Systems

By display system is meant the device which provides the final data to the technician from the nuclear medicine instrument used during the study. The display may be as simple as a needle deflection on a rate meter or as complex as a digital image on an oscilloscope screen. The signals from a detector are first amplified and then subjected to pulse-height analysis. The pulse-height analyzer may be a simple discriminator—an electronic circuit designed to reject very small pulses (noise) and pass every other pulse—or a window, so that only pulses which meet the requirements of an upper and lower discriminator are accepted. In any case, the output of the pulse-height analyzer is usually a pulse of fixed size, as shown in Figure 6-19. These pulses are fed to a display system.

Scalers and scaler-timers.—The pulses from a pulse-height analyzer may be sent to a scaler or scaler-timer combination. A scaler is a device which adds one count to its display system each time a pulse is passed by the pulse-height analyzer. Most scalers have built-in timers so that counts are collected over a specified time period. A typical scaler-timer is shown in Figure 7-10. Such systems are often used for thyroid uptake tests and for all in vitro tests. After radioactivity from a sample or patient is counted, it is necessary to subtract the background count in order to obtain the correct net count in sample or patient. The statistic considerations discussed later in this chapter must be applied to the results of these counting experiments.

Count rate meters.—The pulses from a pulse-height analyzer may be fed to a count rate meter, which reads the number of counts occurring in the detector per minute or per second. Count rate meters are designed to

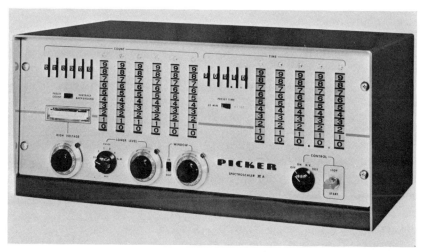

Fig. 7-10.—A typical scaler-timer. Counts are recorded on the left group of scalers, and time (in units of 0.01 minute or 0.1 second) is recorded on the right side. (Courtesy of Picker Corporation, Medical Products Division, Nuclear Department, North Haven, Connecticut.)

average the count rate over a specific period of time called the time constant. Knowledge of the time constant of a rate meter is almost as important as the actual reading of the meter. The effect of the time constant on reading of a count rate meter with two different time constants is shown graphically in Figure 7-11. Note that the short time constant follows the input count rate very well, whereas there is considerable lag in the response of the meter with the long time constant. This means that rapid changes in count rate are not accurately recorded by the count rate meter. When the count rate of pulses from a sample or patient is relatively low, the longer time constant is preferable, since the fluctuations in the

Fig. 7-11.—The effect of short and long time constants on the reading of a rate meter is shown. Changes in input are reflected much more rapidly in the short than in the long time constant.

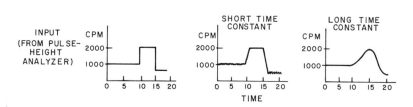

meter reading with a short time constant will be so great as to make the report unmeaningful.

Most rate meters have associated with them a selection switch which allows the rate meter to respond over a very wide range of count rates. When used in scanning systems, the meters have ranges from 300 to over 100,000 counts per minute. When used in survey meters incorporating Geiger-Muller tubes, the count rate meters are also calibrated in radiation exposure units per hour. These survey instruments are usually calibrated for radiation exposure readings with a standard source of radium (^{266}Ra).

Imaging systems.—Thus far, display systems have dealt with the numeric display of data—counts obtained over a specific time interval and recorded on a scaler, or an averaging system which displays counts per minute. The next group of display systems to be discussed provide images of the organ being scanned. All scanning systems provide a dot or tap scan. The actual production of a dot scan will be taken up in detail later, but the mechanism will be discussed here. Marks are placed on heat-sensitive paper in a dot scan or typed on plain white paper in a tap scan. The marks are produced whenever a preselected number of counts has been passed by the pulse-height analyzer. The number of counts required to produce a mark is called the dot factor and may be selected by a rotatable switch on a scanner. Some scanners provide a switch to prevent dots from being recorded unless the count rate is above a certain percentage of full-scale deflection on the count rate meter. The dot factor is usually set to produce between 6 and 10 dots per centimeter on the scan. (The calculation of the dot factor is discussed later in the chapter under the heading Information Density.) The tap factor is usually set to give about 80 taps per centimeter.

In addition to the dot scan, scanners produce an image of the organ being scanned on photographic film. The image is not a photograph of the organ, but a representation of the distribution of the radioactive material in the organ. The film, which is usually 14 inches by 17 inches (a holdover from radiology) is enclosed in a light-tight compartment in the scanner. The film is exposed to a light source, which is a high-speed electronic device which can be turned on and off very rapidly. The brightness of the light source is controlled by the rate meter reading; the brighter the light source, the blacker will be the film at that position.

We have now reviewed all the elements necessary to produce a scanner. Most scanning devices are rectilinear; that is, the path followed by the detector over the patient is as shown in Figure 7-12. The parts of a scanner are assembled schematically in Figure 7-13. The shielded detector, with a collimator in front, is mounted on a rigid beam. The detector

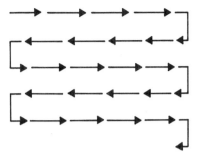

Fig. 7-12.—The path of the detector in rectilinear scanning. The path distance from side to side and the spacing between lines may be varied.

follows a rectilinear path, as indicated in Figure 7-12. High voltage is provided to operate the photomultiplier tube. On the same beam with the detector are mounted the light source and the dot or tap device. Gamma-ray events detected by the scintillation crystal are converted to voltage pulses in the photomultiplier tube. These pulses go to an amplifier and the amplified pulses are fed to the pulse-height analyzer. The output of the pulse-height analyzer goes to two output devices: the dot scan control and the rate meter. The dot scan control sends a signal to the tapper or marker, which places a mark on the scan paper each time a preselected number (the dot factor) of pulses has successfully passed the pulse-height analyzer.

The reading on the rate meter is used to modulate the voltage supplied

Fig. 7-13.—The elements of a rectilinear scanner.

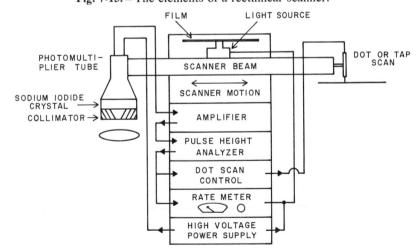

to the light source. When the reading is low, the film exposure is low; the exposure increases to full-film blackness as the rate meter reading increases. Details of setting up a scanner for organ imaging are outlined in Chapter 8.

The mechanism of producing an image with a gamma-ray camera is much different from that of a scanner. When a gamma ray interacts with the large sodium iodide scintillation crystal of a camera, the scintillations are observed by an array (usually 19) of photomultiplier tubes. Naturally, the phototubes directly above the interaction site will receive most of the light, but the others will observe some light also. The pulse output of each of the phototubes in the array is totaled and sent to a pulse-height analyzer which provides an output pulse to a display oscilloscope. Electronically, the crystal is divided into four quadrants, as shown in Figure 7-14. The signals from each of the phototubes are analyzed to determine at what point the gamma occurred in the crystal. The amount of $+x$, $-x$, $+y$, and $-y$ distance from the center of the crystal is measured in a complex circuit called the position analyzer. The position analyzer provides two voltage pulses to the display oscilloscope, one for the x-direction, and one for the y-direction. The display oscilloscope flashes a dot on its screen when a gamma ray meets the requirements of the pulse-height analyzer. The position of the dot depends on the signals from the position analyzer. There is then a one-to-one relationship between the location of a gamma-ray event in the scintillation crystal and

Fig. 7-14.—The electronic circuits in schematic form for a gamma-ray camera. Only five tubes are shown for simplicity.

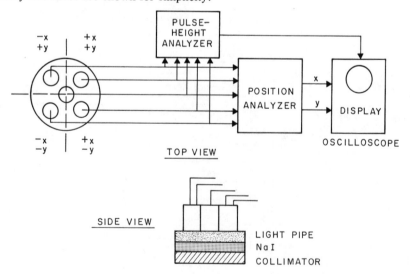

the location of the flash on the display oscilloscope. Usually, a Polaroid or 35 mm. camera is mounted on the display oscilloscope to photograph the dots flashed on the oscilloscope, thus producing a scintiphoto. The product of a diagnostic examination performed with a gamma-ray camera is then a photograph of the sum of a large number of dots produced on the display oscilloscope. There is usually a scaler associated with the camera console which provides a count of the total number of events which have been passed by the pulse-height analyzer. Up to 500,000 counts may be accumulated for a brain scan performed with a gamma-ray camera.

Dynamic Imaging Systems

A variety of electronic data processing (EDP) systems are now available and have been interfaced with all types of nuclear medicine imaging systems including rectilinear scanners and gamma-ray cameras. The uses of EDP systems in nuclear medicine are centered on two principal goals: image enhancement, and recording and analysis of dynamic data. Image enhancement is probably most easily understood in terms of making details of a picture more easily recognizable. For example, the response of a gamma-ray camera may not be uniform over the entire face of the crystal; a computer may then be used to make a point-by-point correction for camera nonuniformity based on a reference picture obtained on a uniform source of activity.

By far the greatest use of EDP systems in nuclear medicine is their application to dynamic studies in which the flow of a radioactively labeled material through or into an organ is recorded as a function of time. Here, a distinction must be made between analogue and digital data. Generally, analogue data have intensities which are proportional to the input. Thus, on a scan, the variation in intensity of the blackness of the film is an analogue of the variation in the amount of radioactive material in the organ being scanned. To convert the analogue signal to digital form means to assign a number to the size of the signal. The number assigned to a digital scan may be simply the number of counts per second over one small area. The results of imaging a simple phantom by both analogue and digital methods are shown in Figure 7-15. Here, the digital record was obtained by using the position signals from a gamma-ray camera; however, rather than using the signals to deflect the dot flashed on the oscilloscope screen, the dots were sorted into a five-by-seven grid of scalers, thus providing the digital record shown.

Dynamic studies may be performed in either analogue or digital fashion. An example of an analogue system would be the taking of a moving picture record of the oscilloscope screen of a gamma-ray camera while a

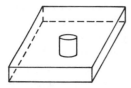

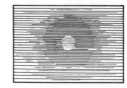

270	260	280	265	268	290	272
279	265	245	219	250		
255	272	230	50	240		
260		225	220	235		
271						

Phantom, filled with radioactive material,except for central cylindrical defect.

Analog image, obtained with rectilear scanner.

Digital image,obtained by sorting position signals from gamma camera into 5 x 7 grid.

Fig. 7-15.—Analogue and digital records obtained on a simple phantom.

radioisotope-labeled material is passing through or being accumulated in an organ. A digital dynamic study could be performed by storing a series of digital images on magnetic disks or tape during an injection of radioactive material. Alternatively, a record of the x- and y-positions of each gamma-ray event detected could be stored sequentially on tape or disk. All of these technics have the advantages that the dynamic study may be played over and over again after the patient has left the nuclear medicine clinic, and the data can·be permanently stored as part of the patient's medical record.

All of medicine is becoming more quantitative in the 1970's, and ability to perform numeric analyses of dynamic studies gives the digital systems a clear advantage over the analogue recording methods in this respect. However, the computers required to perform the analyses are not inexpensive, and the information available from an analogue record may be just as valuable in making a diagnosis.

The EDP systems which have been interfaced with nuclear medicine instrumentation are so varied that a description of their operation and maintenance would require another book to cover all of them adequately. However, most computer systems can perform a number of functions, of which the most important will be discussed here. The mechanism of the technician-computer interaction may be widely different from one EDP system to another, but the actual function is essentially the same in each.

One of the most basic types of dynamic studies is the rate of uptake of a radiopharmaceutical by an organ. Figure 7-16 shows the count rate over the liver as a function of time after intravenous injection of ^{99m}Tc-sulfur colloid. This curve was obtained by selecting a region of interest in one section of the liver (a 4-by-4 grid) and instructing a computer to sum the number of counts per frame in that region as a function of time. Since the ^{99m}Tc-sulfur colloid is removed from the blood and held in the liver, the curve is not surprising. A more complex study involving the

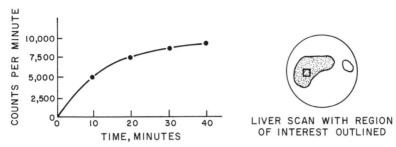

LIVER SCAN WITH REGION
OF INTEREST OUTLINED

Fig. 7-16. — Uptake by the liver of ^{99m}Tc-sulfur colloid as a function of time after injection of the radiopharmaceutical. An area in the liver was selected, and the computer was asked to add up the number of counts per minute in that section as the ^{99m}Tc-sulfur colloid was scavenged and retained by the liver.

flow of ^{99m}Tc (as sodium pertechnetate) through the chambers of the heart is shown in Figure 7-17. Here, the computer has summed the number of counts in the several heart chambers and the lungs to produce the curves shown in the figure. The concentration of the isotope in the heart chambers and lungs can be seen to change very rapidly in just a few seconds.

The two studies outlined here are typical of those performed in nuclear medicine. With the advent of many new radiopharmaceuticals labeled

Fig. 7-17. — A dynamic study involving the flow of ^{99m}Tc through the heart chambers. The scintiphotos show selected portions of the study. The radiopharmaceutical was injected into an arm vein. The areas selected to represent the heart chambers and the lung are shown in the scintiphotos.

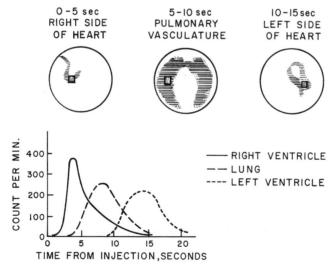

with ^{99m}Tc, the number of organ systems which might be subjected to dynamic studies should increase markedly. The information provided by these dynamic studies will add a new dimension to nuclear medicine — the functional state of organ systems — in addition to their size and shape.

It should be noted that the birth of the specialty of nuclear medicine can be dated from the first evaluation of thyroid function, a dynamic study which measures the uptake of radioactive iodine by the thyroid gland. Here, the uptake is followed for up to several days in order to determine the functional state of the gland. It was not until the development of scintillation counters that the size and shape of the thyroid gland could be determined by means of a rectilinear scan.

Statistics of Counting

All radioactive decay events are random processes. This statement means that in a group of radioactive atoms, it is impossible to state with certainty which atom will decay next. Since random processes can be described only by using statistics, it is necessary to understand some basic statistic principles, especially as applied to nuclear medicine.

The science of statistics deals with the notion of chance: the chance of rain tomorrow, the chance of throwing seven on a pair of dice, or the chance that one measurement of a counting rate is the true or correct value. Statisticians deal with a number scale between zero and one. An event that is certain to occur has a probability of 1.00 or 100%, and an event that is certain never to occur has a probability of 0.00 or 0%. All other events have probabilities between 0.00 and 1.00. Thus, the probability of tossing a head on a single toss of a coin is 0.5, and the probability of drawing an ace from a full deck of 52 cards is 4 of 52, or 0.078. With counting rates, it is desirable to know the accuracy of a count rate (how close to the true value of the count rate the result is) and the probability that the result might be wrong. If a thyroid uptake measurement yields a count rate of 2,500 counts per minute, can anything be said about the accuracy of the result and how far off the result might be? Statistics can provide answers to both of these questions.

In analyzing the results of counting experiments and other random events, statisticians have developed the concept of the standard deviation, represented by the Greek letter sigma (σ). The standard deviation of N counts is simply the square root of N; in equation form,

$$\sigma_N = \sqrt{N}. \qquad (7\text{-}1)$$

Usually, a count is reported with its standard deviation, such as

2,500 ± 50 (N ± σ_N). The count rate (CR) of a sample is given by

$$CR = \frac{N \pm \sqrt{N}}{t} \qquad (7\text{-}2)$$

in which t is the time (in minutes or seconds) over which the count was obtained. For example, if a sample is counted for 10 minutes and 2,500 counts are obtained, the counting rate is 250 ± 5 counts per minute (cpm). If the same number of counts were accumulated in 5 minutes, the count rate would be 500 ± 10 cpm.

The next question that comes to mind is the meaning of the standard deviation. What does σ tell us about the accuracy of the count, and what is the probability that the count may be wrong? It turns out that the value of σ answers these questions. Statistic analysis can show that if a radioactive sample is counted many times, there will be a distribution of results which produces the familiar bell-shaped curve shown in Figure 7-18, the result of counting a sample of radioactive material several hundred times for one-minute intervals. Most of the results cluster around the true value, 2,500 cpm, but there are wide variations. Analysis of the curve of Figure 7-18 shows that 68% of the results are between 2,500 ± 50 (N ± σ_N), and that 95% are between 2,500 ± 100 (N ± 2 σ_N), and 99.7% are between 2,500 ± 150 (N ± 3 σ_N). From these results, we can estimate the accuracy of any count rate measurement. The probability that the correct answer for one measurement is within one standard deviation (N ± σ_N) is 0.68 (about 2 chances of 3); the probability that the correct answer is within two standard deviations (N ± 2 σ_N) is 0.95 (about 19 chances of 20), *etc.*

The standard deviation can also be expressed as a percentage of the total count. Table 7-1 gives the standard deviation values associated

Fig. 7-18.—Results of many counting runs on the same radioactive sample. Several hundred one-minute counts were obtained on this sample which has a true counting rate of 2,500 counts per minute.

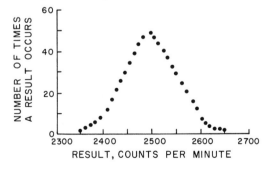

with the total number of observed counts. The standard deviation is independent of the time required to collect the count. It does not matter whether one sample produces 10,000 counts in one minute, whereas another sample must be counted for 20 minutes to acquire 10,000 counts. The standard deviation is the same in both cases: ± 100 counts, or $\pm 1\%$. Of course, the count rates will be much different: $10,000 \pm 100$ cpm for the first sample, and 500 ± 5 cpm for the second.

We now know how to express the count rate and standard deviation for a count. The next problem is to examine the effects of background and to determine how the standard deviation of a background count is to be combined with a sample-plus-background value. The problem is best discussed in terms of an example:

TABLE 7-1.—STANDARD DEVIATIONS ASSOCIATED
WITH A WIDE RANGE OF OBSERVED COUNTS

| | STANDARD DEVIATION | |
COUNTS OBSERVED	Counts	Per cent
10	± 3	± 30.0
20	± 4	± 20.0
50	± 7	± 14.0
100	± 10	± 10.0
200	± 14	± 7.0
500	± 22	± 4.4
1,000	± 32	± 3.2
2,000	± 45	± 2.2
5,000	± 71	± 1.4
10,000	± 100	± 1.0
20,000	± 141	± 0.70
50,000	± 223	± 0.45
100,000	± 316	± 0.32

A well scintillation counter is used to evaluate a Schilling test. The sample-plus-background count is 6,400 in 1.0 minute. The background alone is 1,600 in 1.0 minute. What is the net sample count rate and its standard deviation? Using equation 7-2,

$$\text{Sample} + \text{background } CR = 6,400 \pm 80 \text{ cpm}$$

$$\text{background } CR = 1,600 \pm 40 \text{ cpm.}$$

The net sample count is obviously 4,800 cpm. The standard deviation of the net count is given by:

$$\sigma_{\text{sample}} = \sqrt{(\sigma_{S+B})^2 + (\sigma_B)^2}. \qquad (7\text{-}3)$$

Using this equation, σ_{sample} is found to be ± 89. This is larger than either of the standard deviations of the sample-plus-background alone.

The rule expressed in equation 7-3 is general and may be applied to any sample which must be corrected for background counts.

Resolving Time and Dead Time

Both sodium iodide scintillation detectors and Geiger tubes, together with the amplifiers and pulse-height analyzers associated with them, require a certain amount of time to record and process a pulse. This time is called the dead time or resolving time of the counting system. During the dead time, the counting system cannot process counts and any radiation entering the detector is not counted. This leads to small errors in count rate measurements, but these errors become larger at high count rates.

Geiger-Muller detectors have a dead time of approximately 100 microseconds, whereas scintillation counting systems usually have dead times of about one microsecond. Thus, the dead-time losses are much more severe with G-M tubes. The correct rate for any system can be obtained by means of the equation

$$R = \frac{R^*}{1 - R^* \tau} \tag{7-4}$$

in which R is the corrected count rate, R* is the observed count rate, and τ is the counting system dead time. The units of R* and τ must be complimentary; if R* is in counts per minute, the dead time must be expressed in minutes. Table 7-2 gives the corrected count rates for scintillation and G-M counting systems for various count rates. As seen in the table, significant errors begin to appear with the G-M system at count rates above about 50,000 cpm, although the scintillation system

---

TABLE 7-2.—CORRECTED COUNT RATES FROM VARIOUS COUNTS OBTAINED WITH G-M AND SCINTILLATION SYSTEMS, WITH DEAD TIMES OF 100 μSECONDS AND 2.0 μSECONDS, RESPECTIVELY

OBSERVED COUNT RATE (CPM)	CORRECTED COUNT RATE (CPM) G-M	Scintillation
1,000	1,002	1,000
2,000	2,007	2,000
5,000	5,042	5,002
10,000	10,200	10,004
20,000	20,700	20,007
50,000	54,500	50,040
100,000	115,800	100,200
200,000	300,000	200,660
500,000	3,000,000	500,500
1,000,000	Inoperable	1,036,000

has only small losses even up to 1 million cpm. This is one reason why scintillation detectors have superceded Geiger counters for many applications in nuclear medicine; the count losses become prohibitive at moderately high counting rates with G-M counters. A second principal reason for the preference for the scintillation system is the much greater detection efficiency for gamma rays.

Information Density

Thus far, the discussion in this book has been limited to general concepts of the physics and instrumentation of nuclear medicine. The concept of information density is directly applicable to obtaining high-quality rectilinear scans and scintiphotos from a gamma-ray camera. Briefly, the basic goal of information density is the aquisition of optimum scans and scintiphotos consistent with patient comfort and the amount of time involved in obtaining a scan. A number of studies have shown that the best scans are obtained with an information density of approximately 800 counts per square centimeter (c./cm²). At information densities below 800 c./cm² some information is invariably lost, and above 800 c./cm² there is no significant improvement in scan quality or readability.

The equation for the information density (ID) on a rectilinear scan is

$$ID = \frac{CR}{LS \times SS} \qquad (7\text{-}5)$$

in which CR is the count rate in counts per minute over the organ being scanned, LS is the line spacing in centimeters between successive passes on the scanner, and SS is the scan speed in centimeters per minute. An example of the use of equation 7-5 follows. A liver scan is to be obtained on a patient who has received 1 mCi of ^{99m}Tc. The count rate over the liver is found to be 24,000 cpm. At what scan speed should the rectilinear scanner be operated to obtain an information density of 800 c./cm²? If the line spacing is chosen to be 0.3 cm., substitution in equation 7-5 gives

$$800 \text{ c./cm}^2 = \frac{24{,}000 \text{ cpm}}{0.3 \text{ cm.} \times SS}$$

Solving for SS gives a scanning speed of 100 cpm.

A large number of tables, graphs and charts are available from scanner manufacturers and radiopharmaceutical producers for scan speed settings at various count rates. In some of the newest scanners, all the settings are made automatically by the instrument itself. Since each instrument has its own set of controls for obtaining optimum scans, it would require another book to cover all of them in detail. The technician should refer to the operating manual for the particular instrument being used for detailed instructions on setting the scan controls.

Although not readily apparent, the concept of information density is also applicable to scintiphotos obtained with a gamma-ray camera. The number of counts obtained on a scintiphoto divided by the area of the organ being examined should be approximately 800 c./cm². Thus, for a liver scintiphoto, the area of the liver is approximately 200 cm² (but may be considerably larger or smaller), and the number of counts obtained to produce an information density of 800 c./cm² is about 160,000. For larger organs the number of counts should be increased in direct proportion to the size, and it may be reduced slightly for smaller livers.

The dot or tap factor has been discussed earlier in the chapter. As mentioned earlier, the tap factor is usually set to produce approximately 60 to 100 taps per centimeter. The correct tap factor can be calculated from the maximum count rate over the patient and the scanning speed. The tap factor (TF) is given by

$$TF = \frac{MCR}{TD \times SS} \tag{7-6}$$

in which MCR is the maximum count rate (cpm), TD is the tap density (60 to 100 taps per centimeter), and SS is the scan speed in centimeters per minute.

The dot factor, which is used on instruments which burn a mark on the dot scan, is usually about 10 times larger than the tap factor. Thus, in the liver scan mentioned above with an MCR of 24,000 cpm, the tap factor is 4 if the tap density is 60, and, rounded to the closest dot factor setting, the dot factor is 32.

It must be stressed that the information provided here is only rudimentary and is designed only to provide an insight into the operation of rectilinear scanners and gamma-ray cameras. The best reference for detailed instruction on the operation and maintenance of a nuclear medicine instrument is the manufacturer of the equipment.

SUGGESTED READING

Blahd, W. H. (ed.) *Nuclear Medicine* (2d ed.; New York: McGraw-Hill Book Company, Inc., 1971), Chap. 1.

Hine, G. J. (ed.): *Instrumentation in Nuclear Medicine*, Vol. I (New York: Academic Press, Inc., 1967).

Maynard, C. D.: *Clinical Nuclear Medicine* (Philadelphia: Lea & Febiger, 1969), Chap. 1.

Snell, A. H. (ed.): *Nuclear Instruments and Their Uses*, Vol. I (New York: John Wiley and Sons, Inc., 1962).

STUDY QUESTIONS

1. List the components of a nuclear medicine detection system. Give a brief description of their function.
2. Discuss the similarities and differences between collimators for rectilinear scanners and cameras.
3. What is the reason for using a diverging collimator on a gamma-ray camera?
4. What would happen if a collimator designed for a maximum energy of 200 keV were used for ^{131}I?
5. List the types of display systems used in nuclear medicine instrumentation and the general purpose use of each type.
6. Discuss the effects of long and short time constants on low, medium and high count rates.
7. What is the difference between the dot or tap scan and a photoscan?
8. Discuss the advantages and disadvantages of a gamma-ray camera system as compared to a rectilinear scanner.
9. How are dynamic imaging systems used in nuclear medicine?
10. Calculate the count rate (counts per minute [cpm]) and standard deviation (in cpm and percentages) for the following counting experiments:

COUNTING TIME IN MINUTES	OBSERVED COUNT
1.0	10,000
10.0	10,000
2.5	25,000
10.0	100
4.0	1,000
15.0	3,000

11. Calculate the net count rate in cpm and the standard deviation (cpm and percentages) for the following counting experiments:

SAMPLE PLUS BACKGROUND		BACKGROUND	
COUNT	TIME IN MINUTES	COUNT	TIME IN MINUTES
10,000	1.0	100	1.0
250	1.0	200	1.0
125	1.0	125	1.0
15,000	10.0	1,000	10.0
100,000	100.0	55	1.0

12. Discuss the advantages of sodium iodide scintillation detectors over Geiger counters in terms of the dead time of each detector.
13. What is the meaning of the term information density, and how does it affect the quality of images obtained on nuclear medicine instrumentation?

CHAPTER 8

Clinical Nuclear Medicine

THE PREVIOUS CHAPTERS OF THIS BOOK have been devoted to the physics and instrumentation of nuclear medicine. The goal of all this information is to provide the technician with the background to use the instruments of nuclear medicine to produce diagnostic information concerning a patient's health. The examination of a patient or sample obtained from a patient is the central part of a nuclear medicine technician's work, and the methods and technics used for these examinations are taken up in detail here.

Radiopharmaceuticals

The name "radiopharmaceuticals" is somewhat of a misnomer, since although many of the materials used in nuclear medicine are radioactive, very few of them have any pharmacologic effect. In fact, in the case of ^{99m}Tc, the amount of technetium injected into the patient is about one billionth of a gram (see Chap. 5), and it would be surprising indeed if this amount of ^{99m}Tc produced any effects.

The radiopharmaceutical used in any particular diagnostic examination in nuclear medicine depends on the organ being studied. In the design of radiopharmaceuticals, physiologic response and function of an organ are studied first. For example, liver scanning is performed with colloidal sulfur particles (approximately 10^{-4} cm. in diameter) tagged with ^{99m}Tc because one of the functions of the liver is to remove such particles from the bloodstream. Thus, using this type of radiopharmaceutical, the functional state of the liver (as well as its size and shape) can be determined. Other specific examples will be provided in later sections.

Radiopharmaceuticals are presently available from a number of pharmaceutical manufacturers who provide the materials in sterile, pyrogen-free state. The requirements for sterility and freedom from pyrogens are given in the United States Pharmacopeia (USP). Sterility means to be free of disease-causing organisms. Freedom from pyrogens means that the radiopharmaceutical will not produce a fever after intravenous injection, since this is the main route of administration of radiopharmaceuticals in nuclear medicine.

97

In the United States, the acquisition, storage, and use of any radioactive materials containing nuclear reactor-produced isotopes are presently under the control of the Atomic Energy Commission (AEC), except in those states ("agreement states") which have taken over control of radioactive materials under agreements with the federal AEC. The prerequisite for the operation of a nuclear medicine clinic is a license from the AEC or from the state licensing authority.

Control of radiopharmaceuticals had been with the AEC since its establishment, but in 1971 this control was taken over by the Food and Drug Administration (FDA). It appears that isotope licensing will still be required, but the safety and efficacy of radiopharmaceuticals will be under the control of the FDA. In addition, any hospital or medical center that allows use of radiopharmaceuticals must have a radioisotope committee to pass on the use of these radioactive materials. This system of checks and balances has served nuclear medicine well, providing for orderly growth of the specialty with adequate safeguards for the patients served.

Patient Care

As a technician, you will be the patient's main contact in nuclear medicine. Your responsibility to the patient is large, demanding and real. The patient is in your care, and you will be responsible for his well-being while he is in the nuclear medicine clinic. Although most of the diagnostic examinations in nuclear medicine are passive in the sense that the patient is not subject to manipulation or surgery, there are two areas in which special care must be taken. The first is patient identification—always verify the identity of a patient before doing anything else. All hospitals now provide wrist or ankle bands for patients, so it is a simple matter to identify even an unconscious patient. The second item to be especially concerned with is the amount and identity of the isotope to be given to the patient. It is an excellent habit to check and recheck dose calculations and the vial from which isotopes are dispensed.

Many states in the United States have laws prohibiting anyone except a licensed physician from injecting drugs intravenously. Since most radiopharmaceuticals are administered intravenously, these laws require the injections to be made by a licensed physician. However, many hospitals have obtained exemptions from these laws for special cases, such as the starting of intravenous medications by trained nurses (IV teams), and the intravenous injection of radiopharmaceuticals by trained nuclear medicine technicians. If you are permitted to administer radiopharmaceuticals, the above two points become even more important, and two additional factors must be considered: (1) you must insist on a written request from a physician that the examination be performed, and (2) you must have the patient's consent to administer the radiopharmaceutical. Without a written request and the patient's consent, the administration of radiopharmaceuticals may result in a lawsuit with you as the defendant. It is not your job to force the patient to submit to an examination he does not want; however, it is permissible to attempt to explain the procedure to him in realistic terms in an effort to obtain medically useful information.

Almost all examinations done in nuclear medicine require that the patient be lying down, usually on a stretcher. Ambulatory patients should be assisted in getting on or off the stretcher. Inpatients who are too ill to travel by wheelchair should arrive at the clinic already on stretchers. Every effort should be made to ensure the patient's comfort — use clean linen over stretcher pads, provide pillows, *etc.* Safety straps should be used on all patients, and stretcher rails should be up whenever the examination permits.

Keep the patient reassured and informed on what will occur during the examination, but do not divulge to the patient medical information obtained before, during or after the procedure. Persistent questions from the patient usually indicate anxiety concerning his diagnosis or prognosis, but it is still not permissible to give him any medical information — leave this to the patient's physician. You should give the patient a realistic estimate of the time required to perform the examination and remind him that his cooperation will be required to produce interpretable results.

An emergency tray should be maintained and periodically inventoried in the clinic. The tray should include drugs to combat serious allergic reactions, blood pressure-measuring system, stethoscope, a tracheostomy set, emergency oxygen, and a suction pump. A physician should be present in the clinic at all times to meet the inevitable medical emergencies which occur.

Many examinations in nuclear medicine require the placement of anatomic markings on the dot scan. For outpatients, this may require removal of some clothing, especially for liver scans, since most physicians prefer to palpate the liver while the patient is under the scanning device. Also, for any scan or scintiphoto, it will be necessary to avoid absorption of gamma radiation by bulky or dense objects between the organ being scanned and the radiation detector. For these tests, the patient is given a hospital gown and covered with a sheet.

In Vivo Examinations

These examinations include all nuclear medicine procedures performed that involve the injection or ingestion of radioactive materials into a patient. A radiopharmaceutical is administered to a patient and its rate of uptake, location of uptake, passage through, or excretion by an organ system is determined.

THYROID STUDIES

The use of radioactive iodine for the evaluation of the function of the thyroid gland was the beginning of nuclear medicine in the 1930s, and the simple radioactive iodine uptake (RAI uptake) test is still in general use, although its usefulness in diagnosing thyroid illness is declining somewhat with the advent of other in vitro tests for evaluating thyroid function.

The thyroid gland is located in the lower part of the neck between the Adam's apple and the sternal notch. The gland is nearly symmetric, with one lobe on each side of the neck; the lobe size increases with age, assuming an over-all length of 4 to 7 cm. in adults. The thyroid gland produces thyroid hormone, which contains iodine. The rate of uptake of radioactive iodine provides a measure of the functional state of the gland, since it cannot distinguish between normal stable iodine and ^{131}I and incorporates both into thyroid hormone. The function of the gland may be awry because of disease of the thyroid gland itself (primary thyroid illness) or because of primary disease in the pituitary, which releases thyroid-stimulating hormone (TSH) in response to levels of thyroid hormone in the bloodstream (secondary thyroid disease).

The RAI uptake test measures the amount of radioactive iodine taken up by the thyroid gland after ingestion of sodium iodide-^{131}I. This radiopharmaceutical is usually given as a drink, although some manufacturers provide calibrated amounts of ^{131}I in capsules. If only an uptake test is being done, as little as 5 μCi of ^{131}I will provide accurate results. Up to 100 μCi of ^{131}I are given if a scan is to be done with ^{131}I; however, in most clinics ^{99m}Tc is used for thyroid scanning. Other iodine isotopes, notably ^{125}I and ^{123}I, have been proposed for use in RAI uptake studies, but both have serious deficiencies. ^{125}I emits only low-energy (28 keV) x-rays; the absorption of these photons can differ from patient to patient. The ^{123}I can be produced only in an accelerator, and is not generally available.

A standard containing the same amount of ^{131}I is prepared and its radioactivity is counted at the same time the radioactivity emitted by the patient is counted. The standard is usually prepared at the same time as the drinks and is placed in some sort of phantom device to simulate the patient's neck. The phantom may be a quite elaborate affair or may be as simple as a grooved block of wood onto which the bottled standard is placed. The uptake is always measured at 24 hours after ingestion, but many physicians also determine the uptake at 2 and 6 hours.

A sodium iodide scintillation detector is used to count the 364-keV gamma rays of [131]I. The detector crystal is shielded and collimated, as shown in Figure 8-1. A positioning rod is attached to the detector to provide reproducible counting conditions for each sample counted. The pulse-height analyzer is adjusted so that only the 364-keV gamma rays of ^{131}I are detected. This adjustment is often called peaking and can be done at least two ways. The first method involves setting the photomultiplier tube high voltage at some predetermined value, usually between 900 and 1,000 volts. Then, using a standard source of ^{131}I, the lower-level discriminator is adjusted (with a constant window) to obtain the maximum count rate. A typical set of values obtained during a peaking operation using this technic is given in Table 8-1.

The second method of peaking the instrument is to select a lower-level discriminator setting, again with a constant window, and then to vary the photomultiplier tube high voltage. The lower-level discriminator is usually a multiturn potentiometer which can be read to three significant figures. One method of selecting the lower-level discriminator is to dial in the gamma-ray energy—in this case, 364 keV. Counts of a standard source of ^{131}I are then obtained at a number of high-voltage settings. A typical set of data obtained by this technic is also shown in Table 8-1. Both methods accomplish the same result—the detector system will count only gamma rays having an energy close to 364 keV. Gamma rays that undergo Compton scattering in the patient or detector and thus deposit less energy in the detector are not counted.

After peaking the detection system, the uptake of radioactive iodine can be measured. Position the detector vertically over the patient's neck with the positioning rod just touching the skin over the gland. Make sure the patient is lying flat without a pillow so that the gland can be viewed without obstruction. Count for one minute. This count (C_N) represents

Fig. 8-1.—A radioactive iodine uptake counting system.

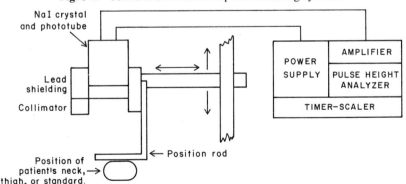

TABLE 8-1.—RESULTS OBTAINED IN THE PEAKING OF A RADIOACTIVE IODINE
UPTAKE SYSTEM BY TWO METHODS, USING A 10 μCi SOURCE OF ^{131}I

CONSTANT HIGH VOLTAGE (1,200 VOLTS); WINDOW SET AT 100 PHU*		CONSTANT LOWER LEVEL DISCRIMINATOR SETTING OF 360 PHU, AND CONSTANT WINDOW (100 PHU)	
Lower level discriminator setting, PHU	Counts per Minute	High Voltage	Counts per Minute
100	6,197	1,080	271
150	6,556	1,100	1,174
200	6,332	1,120	635
250	6,681	1,140	610
300	8,583	1,180	8,895
350	12,971	1,200	14,457
375	14,759	1,220	9,552
400	14,124	1,240	5,631
425	10,343	1,260	3,842

*PHU = pulse height units.

the ^{131}I in the gland, plus any ^{131}I which may be in the surrounding tissue or blood, plus background. The problem now is to separate the ^{131}I counts in the thyroid gland from the background and surrounding tissue counts. There is no method to solve this problem exactly. One technic is to obtain a second count over the patient's thigh, being careful to position the detector well away from the bladder, since ^{131}I is excreted in the urine. The detector is positioned at the standard distance, just touching the skin of the thigh, and a second one-minute count is obtained and designated C_T, the thigh count. This represents the ^{131}I in an amount of tissue and blood which is roughly equivalent to those of the neck, plus background counts. The patient may now leave. Next, position the detector over the phantom containing the ^{131}I standard and count for one minute to obtain C_S, which represents the ^{131}I in the standard plus background counts. Finally, remove the phantom from in front of the detector and count the background for one minute, giving C_B. The percentage of radioactive iodine uptake is then given by the equation

$$RAI \text{ uptake } \% = \frac{(C_N - C_T)\ 100}{C_S - C_B}. \tag{8-1}$$

Twenty-four hour uptake values vary from place to place around the world, depending on the amount of dietary iodine available from natural (salt, seafood) or artificial sources (iodized salt), so it is impossible to set normal limits on uptake values which will be universally applicable. Most nuclear medicine clinics have established uptake values which are considered normal for the area. Even these "local" normal values have been found to change with time, as the dietary habits of a population change or iodized salt becomes available.

Although the RAI uptake measures the function of the thyroid gland, it is often necessary to obtain a picture of the size and shape of the gland in order to evaluate other thyroid diseases. The presence of a palpable nodule on or near the thyroid gland is probably the most common reason for referral of a patient for a thyroid scan. This means that it is important for the technician to obtain anatomic markings on the scan. Usually, the thyroid cartilage and sternal notch are indicated, together with an outline of the gland, if palpable, and any palpable nodules. Thyroid scans are usually done on a rectilinear scanner for these reasons, although a gamma-ray camera with a pinhole collimator can also be used.

At the present time, both ^{131}I (as sodium iodide, NaI) and ^{99m}Tc (as sodium pertechnetate, $NaTcO_4$) are used for thyroid scanning. If ^{131}I is used, the uptake drink is usually 100 μCi of ^{131}I, and the radioiodine taken up by the gland is used for scanning. If ^{99m}Tc is employed, between 1 and 5 mCi of ^{99m}Tc is administered intravenously. The amount of ^{99m}Tc given depends on the result of thyroid uptake of radioactive iodine (^{99m}Tc as the ion TcO_4^- is taken up by the thyroid gland in amounts roughly proportional to ^{131}I; however, the ^{99m}Tc is not incorporated into thyroid hormone). If the ^{131}I uptake is below 10%, 5 mCi of ^{99m}Tc would be given, whereas patients with ^{131}I uptake values above 50% would receive 1 mCi. Patients with intermediate uptake values are given appropriate amounts of ^{99m}Tc.

Thyroid scanning using ^{131}I is best done 24 hours after administration of the ^{131}I drink, but ^{99m}Tc scans should be done within one hour of the time of injection. The patient is positioned supine (lying face up) on a stretcher under the scanner. A pillow under the patient's shoulders may help to throw the neck forward, and keep the chin from being hit by the scanner as it moves back and forth.

Rectilinear scanners are also peaked in the same manner as described in the previous section. Recently, scanner manufacturers have added push buttons to select the photopeaks of the most commonly used gamma-emitting radionuclides. Older instruments are provided with a howler, which is a speaker connected to the rate meter of the instrument. The higher the count rate, the higher the pitch of the howler. The patient can be used as a source of radioactivity to peak the machine. Fit the detector with a "fine" collimator and position it over the area of the thyroid gland. Set the lower-level discriminator and window of the pulse-height analyzer for the gamma-ray energy of the isotope being used (140 keV for ^{99m}Tc, 364 keV for ^{131}I), and vary the detector voltage until the count rate reaches a maximum, as determined by listening to the howler or observing the rate meter. Alternatively, the voltage may be set at a predetermined value (about 1,000 volts) and the lower-level discriminator and window settings adjusted to maximize the count rate.

After peaking the scanner, the patient and stretcher should be positioned so that the scan will all fit on the 14 by 17 inch film. (This positioning is not so critical for thyroid scanning, but is very important for rectilinear scanning of larger organs.) Move the detector head over the thyroid region until the highest count rate is observed. This procedure is called finding the hot spot. The light-source voltage is then adjusted to produce maximum film darkening with the detector in this position. Other instrument settings (scan speed, line spacing, dot or tap factor, *etc.*) are made at this time, but will not be covered here because scanners produced by different manufacturers differ widely in their setups. Refer to the instrument's manual for detailed information on other instrument controls and their operation.

Remind the patient of the requirement to remain immobile during the scan, pull the film slide and start the scanner. Take a few minutes to observe the operation and scan the control knobs to make sure the settings are correct. The normal thyroid gland should be scanned from one side of the neck to the other, and from above the Adam's apple (thyroid cartilage) to below the sternal notch, but extensions above and below these points are not uncommon; make sure you are getting a scan of the entire thyroid gland by checking the dot scan. When the scan is completed, turn the scanner off and replace the film slide. Position the detector over the thyroid cartilage and mark that point on the dot scan. Also mark the sternal notch, any palpable nodules, and outline the gland if possible. These marks are transferred to the film with a marking pencil

Fig. 8-2. – Rectilinear scans of the thyroid gland. The sternal notch is marked on both scans and the thyroid cartilage marking may be seen at the top of the right scan. Scan on right also shows a cold nodule.

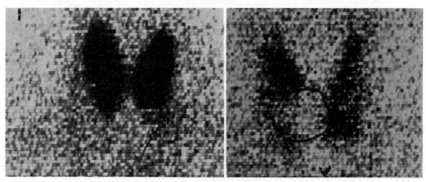

after development of the film. A positive method of identifying dot and film scans is indispensable. The dot scan should be marked with the patient's name, the date, and important instrument settings (hot spot, count rate, scan speed, light-source voltage, collimator used, isotope used for scan, *etc.*). A rubber stamp may be useful, with spaces for entering the appropriate information.

Typical thyroid scans are shown in Figure 8-2. It should be remembered that scans are not pictures like photographs or radiographs, but a representation of the distribution of radioactive material in the organ scanned.

The thyroid uptake and scan examinations may be supplemented by one or more in vitro tests of thyroid function. These tests are discussed in the section under in vitro studies.

Brain and Cerebrospinal Fluid Studies

Brain scanning with ^{99m}Tc (as sodium pertechnetate, $NaTcO_4$) has probably been the making of the specialty of nuclear medicine. This examination provides invaluable information with a minimum of risk to the patient. The examination requires one intravenous injection of several millicuries of radioactive material and the patient's cooperation in remaining still while the scan is being performed. The alternative to brain scanning at the present time is cerebral angiography, which involves injecting a radiopaque dye into the carotid arteries and taking many x-ray photographs of the flow of dye as it traverses the blood supply of the brain. This procedure is not without risk, and the simple and elegant brain scan is a very attractive alternative.

It should be made clear at the outset that brain scanning cannot be used to identify a brain lesion positively as a tumor or any other specific condition, although other clinical data may make one diagnosis more favored than another. Brain scanning with ^{99m}Tc utilizes one of the relatively mysterious functions of brain tissue, the so-called blood-brain barrier. Under normal conditions, the blood-brain barrier acts to exclude most of the ionic components of the blood from entering brain tissue. The barrier leaks when the brain has been subjected to any of a large number of pathologic conditions: tumor (primary or metastatic), cerebral vascular accident (CVA, or stroke), cysts, or subdural hemorrhage. Thus, the normal brain scan will show essentially no activity in the region where brain tissue is located, whereas an abnormal scan will show where radioactive material has leaked past the blood-brain barrier. However, the abnormal scan usually cannot provide any information about the nature of the lesion causing the blood-brain barrier to leak.

The brain scan study usually begins with the administration of a drink containing a water solution of a compound such as sodium perchlorate ($NaClO_4$), although other materials have been recommended from time to time. The perchlorate ion (ClO_4^-) acts chemically like the pertechnetate ion (TcO_4^-) in the body, and especially in a region of the brain called the choroid plexus. Ordinarily, the $^{99m}TcO_4^-$ would be secreted by the choroid plexus and would produce a "hot" area in the brain scan which can mask a pathologic condition or be mistaken for such a condition. An example of the effects of the administration of perchlorate is shown in Figure 8-3, scintiphotos of the brain of a patient taken with and without prior administration of sodium perchlorate. Usually, 500 mg. of $NaClO_4$ in a syrup designed to mask its unpleasant taste is given orally to adult patients at least 15 minutes before ^{99m}Tc is given intravenously. The amount of $NaClO_4$ should be reduced proportionately (by weight) for children and young adults.

At some medical centers, perchlorate, atropine and the ^{99m}Tc are all administered together by intravenous injection. The purpose of the atropine is to reduce secretion of $^{99m}TcO_4^-$ in the salivary glands, which can show up as a hot area in the vertex view of the brain. The administration of both these drugs requires the direction and supervision of a physician. For an obtunded patient or one who cannot be persuaded to drink the sodium perchlorate solution, ^{99m}Tc-DTPA may be injected intravenously instead of ^{99m}Tc as sodium pertechnetate. The ^{99m}Tc-DTPA is more fully described in the Renal Studies section; this radiopharmaceutical is

Fig. 8-3. — ^{99m}Tc brain scintiphotos obtained on the same patient. Scintiphoto on left was obtained without prior administration of sodium perchlorate ($NaClO_4$). Scintiphoto on right was obtained 2 days later, with 500 mg. of $NaClO_4$ administered 30 minutes before injection of ^{99m}Tc. The secretion of ^{99m}Tc by the choroid plexus is effectively blocked.

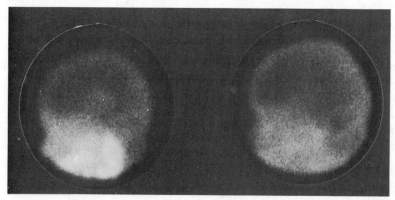

not secreted by the choroid plexus, but is cleared fairly rapidly via the kidneys, so delayed scans are not possible.

The amount of ^{99m}Tc administered for a brain scan is usually 10 mCi for an adult, with proportionately smaller doses for children and young adults. With the widespread use of the gamma-ray camera in many nuclear medicine clinics, it has become practical to obtain a "flow" study by injecting the ^{99m}Tc intravenously while the patient is under the gamma-ray camera. The flow study is obtained by photographing the oscilloscope display screen as the radioactive material rises in the carotid arteries (the main blood supply to the head and brain) and travels through the vascular bed of the brain. With a Polaroid camera, eight pictures can each be exposed for one second or so. This procedure requires a fair amount of manual dexterity in pulling the films, and is also quite expensive (eight Polaroid photos cost approximately $2.50). One much less expensive alternative is to use a 35-mm. camera and an automatic exposure-film advance system, which is available from a number of nuclear medicine instrument manufacturers. A second alternative is to record the flow on magnetic tape in either an analogue or digital mode for later playback. A brain blood-flow study is shown in Figure 8-4; this was obtained with a 35-mm. camera system.

For the flow study and the anterior-posterior (AP) view of the brain, the patient is in a supine position with his head under the gamma-ray camera. Usually a low-energy, straight-hole collimator is used. The proper position is shown in Figure 8-5*A*. Note that the camera head should be tilted slightly in order to "look into" the brain. Although the usual flow study is performed with the patient in the anterior-posterior position, the suspected pathologic condition in a particular patient may

Fig. 8-4. — A brain blood-flow study obtained with a 35-mm. camera and an automatic exposure-film advance system. Photographs were taken of the display oscilloscope of a gamma-ray camera. The stop-motion pictures show equal flow of blood to both hemispheres of the brain.

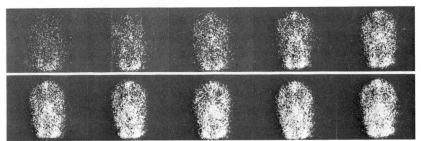

dictate that this part of the examination be done with the camera in one of the other positions shown in Figure 8-5. The correct position should be indicated by the referring physician.

The four- or five-view brain scan (anterior-posterior, posterior-anterior, two lateral views and an optional view) is started not earlier than 30 minutes after the injection of ^{99m}Tc. Some types of tumors will not show an increased amount of activity at this time, and a delayed scan may be requested.

The positioning of the patient's head during brain scanning is very important. The head should be placed so that the gamma-ray camera will

Fig. 8-5. — Patient positions for brain scanning with gamma-ray camera.

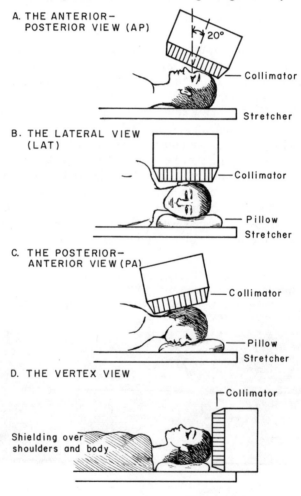

A. THE ANTERIOR–
POSTERIOR VIEW (AP)

20°

Collimator

Stretcher

B. THE LATERAL VIEW
(LAT)

Collimator

Pillow
Stretcher

C. THE POSTERIOR–
ANTERIOR VIEW (PA)

Collimator

Pillow
Stretcher

D. THE VERTEX VIEW

Collimator

Shielding over
shoulders and body

look into the brain in a symmetric fashion. Imagine a plane passing through the patient's head, dividing the brain into left and right sides; the collimator face should be located at a right angle to this plane for the anterior-posterior, posterior-anterior and vertex views, and parallel to this plane for the lateral views. A second plane along the line from eyebrow to ear canal will also be helpful in positioning. This line runs just below the bone structure supporting the base of the brain. In the anterior-posterior, posterior-anterior and lateral views, the camera collimator should be perpendicular to this plane, and the collimator should be parallel to this plane for the vertex view.

Because of the nature of brain scanning, most of the counts collected in a scintiphoto or scan will come from areas that are not actually in the brain. The counts come from ^{99m}Tc circulating in the peripheral vascular bed (scalp and facial vessels), the main venous channels in the brain, and the ^{99m}Tc that has been secreted in saliva (Fig. 8-6). Another problem with brain scanning with the gamma-ray camera is that no depth vision is provided by the collimators; all of the counts originating in the superficial vessels of the head are detected and counted, so they appear on the scintiphoto and degrade the image somewhat. In order to obtain a scintiphoto of diagnostic quality, it is necessary to acquire at least 300,000 counts on the scintiphoto; many clinics routinely obtain 500,000 counts. A marker button containing about 10 μCi of either ^{57}Co (half-life of 270 days, with a gamma ray of 122 kev) or ^{144}Ce (half-life of 285 days, with a gamma ray of 134 kev) should be used to identify the right side

Fig. 8-6.—Brain scintiphotos (*top row*) and rectilinear scans (*bottom row*) showing distribution of ^{99m}Tc in the head. From left to right, the views are anterior-posterior, posterior-anterior, lateral and vertex.

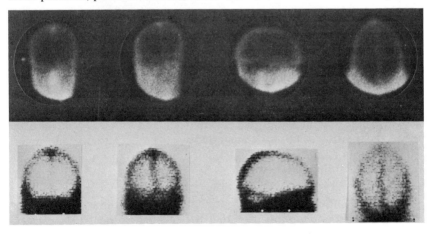

of the head in anterior-posterior, posterior-anterior and vertex views.

Although brain scanning with the gamma-ray camera usually involves the immobilization of the patient and rotation of the camera head itself to meet the position criteria mentioned above, the use of a rectilinear scanner for brain scanning makes many more demands upon the technician and the patient. The detector in the rectilinear scanner is normally operated in the vertical position. The patient must be moved to the correct position and then immobilized so that the face of the collimator is in the same position relative to the patient as mentioned above for the gamma-ray camera. The hot spot for all views is usually located over the apex region of the sagittal sinus, a large venous vessel that drains the brain and runs from roughly the top of the head to the back of the head, as indicated in the scans of Figure 8-6. Brain scanning with a rectilinear scanner usually requires that the contrast enhancement feature of the scanner be used during scanning. Contrast enhancement, when applied to regions in which the count rate differences between adjacent areas are small and correspond to small differences in the range of film darkening, as shown in Figure 8-7, increases the distinction between light and dark areas, thereby allowing better diagnostic accuracy.

Before scanning, the scan speed and other instrument controls should be set as indicated by the manufacturer. One great advantage of rectilinear scanners over cameras is that the former use focused collimators. When properly positioned, the rectilinear scanner is focused in the center of the hemisphere of the brain in lateral views, and several inches inside the skull in the anterior-posterior and posterior-anterior views. In this manner, ^{99m}Tc in the peripheral blood vessels is not in the focal plane of the collimator and so is not detected with high efficiency. This means that the scan is somewhat "cleaner" than the camera-produced scintiphoto. However, this positive aspect of rectilinear scanning is somewhat negated by the increased amount of time required for scanning—about 20 minutes per view for a scanner as opposed to 3 to 5 minutes for the camera.

The dot scan should be marked with the patient's name and other information indicated earlier in the discussion on thyroid scanning: instrument settings, date, view, *etc.* Anatomic landmarks (eyes on anterior-posterior and lateral views, ear canal on lateral view) should also be made on the dot scan and transferred to the film after development. Note that the rectilinear scan provides a full-size representation of the organ scanned; this information can be invaluable to a surgeon contemplating brain surgery.

Brain scanning with ^{99m}Tc can produce several technical hot or cold spots on scans and scintiphotos that the technician must be aware of.

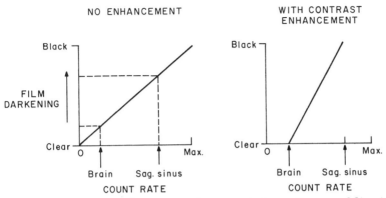

Fig. 8-7.—The concept of contrast enhancement. A small range of film darkening is expanded to cover the whole region from clear to black. In a brain scan, this would lead to scans of good diagnostic quality; however, areas with count rates higher than those in the sagittal sinus would be overexposed. These overexposed regions are not in the diagnostic areas, but well below the brain.

Since ^{99m}Tc (as NaTcO$_4$) is actively secreted in perspiration and saliva and in the stomach, there can be a serious contamination problem for a patient who has vomited or expectorated. A small amount of ^{99m}Tc in the hair will show up as a hot spot. Scalp bumps and lacerations may show increased activity of ^{99m}Tc, producing a hot spot. Holding the patient's head tightly can produce a cold spot in gamma-ray camera views because local scalp circulation may be cut off. Hands and arms must not be in view of the scanner or camera; the activity circulating there will show up. In the vertex view, the patient should be provided with a lead apron which covers the upper body and shoulders to prevent radiation from these areas from reaching the detector (Fig. 8-5*D*).

Another important nuclear medicine procedure involving the head and brain is the cerebrospinal fluid (CSF) scan, sometimes called radioisotope cisternography. This fluid bathes the brain and spinal cord and protects these vital structures from shock and injury. The fluid is produced mainly in the choroid plexus and circulates throughout the ventricles and the outer surfaces of the brain. Blockage of fluid circulation can lead to hydrocephalus, and suspicion of this condition is probably the principal reason for requesting the scan. Human serum albumin (HSA) tagged with ^{131}I—or radioiodinated serum albumin (RISA)—is used for the study. For adults, about 100 μCi of RISA is injected into the cerebrospinal fluid, usually in the lumbar spine region. Smaller amounts are used for children and young adults. This injection should be administered only by a physician well-trained in performing spinal taps under aseptic conditions. The RISA should have the highest possible specific activity (microcuries of ^{131}I per milligram of HSA). This radiopharmaceutical, when injected into the CSF, often causes aseptic meningitis, and appropriate medical support should be available to deal with this problem.

Under normal conditions, the RISA will diffuse up the spinal column into the basal cisterns, through the subarachnoid paths and sylvian fissures to the superior longitudinal sinus. Most of the injected RISA activity will appear in the head in 12 to 24 hours. Scans or scintiphotos are taken at various times after injection, usually at about 2, 4, 12, 24, and sometimes as late as 48 hours.

Rectilinear scanning of CSF studies usually requires two views which are quite similar to ^{99m}Tc brain scans—an anterior-posterior view and one lateral view. The scanner should be "peaked" with ^{131}I. The count rate is likely to be quite low, not more than 3,000 counts per minute, so that the scanning speed will be low, and the study can easily require more than 30 minutes per view. Anatomic markings (eyes, nose, ears, mouth) should be recorded on the dot scan with pertinent patient and instrument settings (Fig. 8-8).

CSF studies can also be obtained with a gamma-ray camera, using a high-energy collimator. The camera should also be "peaked" with a source of ^{131}I, so that only the 364-keV gamma rays of ^{131}I are detected. At least 50,000 counts should be collected for each anterior-posterior and lateral view. A marker button containing about 10 μCi of ^{133}Ba (which

Fig. 8-8.—Normal cerebrospinal fluid scans. *Top row* shows 4-hour views; *bottom row,* 22-hour scans.

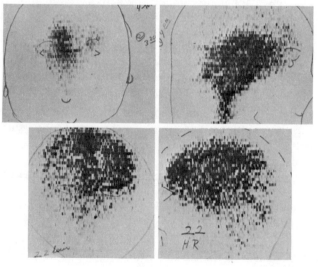

has a gamma ray at 363 keV and a half-life of 7.2 years) can be used to identify the right side of the patient's head in the anterior-posterior view and the front of the head in the lateral view (Fig. 8-8).

In some patients, there may be no detectable radioactivity in the patient's head. This can result from blockage of flow in the spinal region, but is more often caused by injection of the RISA into regions other than the CSF fluid space. If there are no counts in the head region, move the detector or patient and count over the lumbar spine region; a single spot of activity in this area usually indicates an improper injection. These findings should be reported immediately.

LIVER, SPLEEN, BONE MARROW AND PANCREAS

The liver and speen are abdominal organs which can be visualized with the same radiopharmaceutical, and the pancreas is included here because this organ usually requires a liver scan in order to make the pancreas scan diagnostically useful. As with many other nuclear medicine procedures, basic physiologic functions are utilized to concentrate the radiopharmaceutical in the liver, spleen and pancreas. For liver and spleen scans, the radiopharmaceutical used is normally a material called technetium sulfur colloid (TSC) which can be purchased as a sterile, pyrogen-free preparation on a daily basis from radiopharmaceutical manufacturers, or prepared in the clinic using a kit manufactured by one of a number of drug houses. The colloid is prepared by precipitating technetium sulfide (probably Tc_2S_7) onto colloidal sulfur; both Tc_2S_7 and colloidal sulfur are produced in situ by boiling an acidified solution of sodium thiosulfate. The size of the colloid particle obtained by means of this reaction is about 1 μ (10^{-4} cm.). Suspensions of the colloid in water have a milky white, opalescent character. The suspension is stabilized by neutralization with sodium hydroxide containing a sodium salt to produce a buffered solution.

Another colloidal material, colloidal gold containing ^{198}Au, is sometimes used if ^{99m}Tc-sulfur colloid is not available. The ^{198}Au-colloid must be purchased from a radiopharmaceutical manufacturer in sterile, pyrogen-free form. The particle size is much smaller than the ^{99m}Tc preparation, and very little (less than 1%) of the ^{198}Au-colloid is sequestered by the spleen in normal patients; this is in marked contrast to the up to 5% of ^{99m}Tc-sulfur colloid usually captured by the spleen. The radiation dose to the liver is quite high—4 rads for the usual 100 μCi usually injected. Because of the high radiation dose, the use of ^{198}Au has generally declined since the introduction of the ^{99m}Tc-sulfur colloid in the late 1960's.

A number of other colloidal compounds of ^{99m}Tc have been developed for liver scanning; it seems likely that ^{99m}Tc-sulfur colloid will be displaced in its turn by another ^{99m}Tc compound which is not retained indefinitely by the liver.

The colloidal particles, tagged with a radioactive marker of ^{99m}Tc or ^{198}Au, are removed from the bloodstream by groups of cells called reticuloendothelial (RE) cells. The RE cells are found in the liver, spleen and bone marrow. The exact mechanism of removal of colloidal particles by RE cells need not concern us here, but their location is important in the acquisition and interpretation of liver scans. There appears to be a sequence of destruction of the RE system that can be followed by scanning with tagged colloidal particles: the main RE function shifts from liver to spleen to bone marrow in several common liver diseases including cirrhosis and hepatitis. Thus, a shift in the concentration of tagged colloidal particles from liver to spleen to bone marrow occurs in these diseases.

A liver-scanning agent which does not utilize the RE function of the liver is ^{131}I-labeled rose bengal. This material is concentrated in the polygonal cells of the liver, and the material was originally used as a radiopaque dye for liver x-radiography. When labeled with ^{131}I, it is sometimes used for liver scanning. Rose bengal is normally excreted by the liver through the gallbladder and biliary tract into the small intestine; at the present time, ^{131}I-rose bengal is used chiefly to obtain information regarding the degree of obstruction of the biliary tract.

As is the case with brain scans, the abnormal liver or spleen scan cannot usually be interpreted as being caused by one particular disease process. Defects in the liver or spleen are observed as negative defects—places where the RE function (or polygonal cell function for ^{131}I-rose bengal) has been diminished or destroyed—so no radioactivity is detected.

The amounts of radioactivity administered to the patient depend on the radiopharmaceutical used and the size of the patient. Values for the three radiopharmaceuticals are given in Table 8-2. All three are administered intravenously and are rapidly concentrated by the liver (and spleen and marrow for the colloids). Visualization by rectilinear scanner or camera may be started in 15 to 20 minutes, or earlier if ^{131}I-rose bengal is the material used to obtain a liver scan. (The excretion via gallbladder occurs rapidly, and this may interfere with the interpretation of the scan).

At least two views of the liver, anterior and lateral, are obtained. A posterior view is required to visualize the spleen well and is sometimes used for the liver scan. For the anterior view, the patient is placed supine on a stretcher after removal of clothing covering the abdomen (recover the patient with a sheet). The scanner collimator should be placed

TABLE 8-2.—AMOUNTS OF LIVER-SCANNING AGENTS
ADMINISTERED TO ADULT PATIENTS AND THE GAMMA-RAY
ENERGY OF EACH AGENT

RADIOPHARMACEUTICAL	INTRAVENOUS DOSE* (μCi)	GAMMA-RAY ENERGY (keV)
^{99m}Tc-Sulfur colloid	1,000 – 3,000	140
^{198}Au-colloid	100 – 200	412
^{131}I-Rose bengal	100 – 200	364

*Adult dose; this should be scaled down for children and young adults.

so that the focal depth is at least 2 inches below the skin surface. The instrument should be peaked for the correct gamma-ray energy (listed in Table 8-2). Center the patient under the scanner so that both liver and spleen can be visualized on a single view. (This is sometimes impossible with larger patients; if this is the case, concentrate on the liver and use a posterior view to visualize the spleen). After obtaining the hot spot, set the instrument controls as indicated by the manufacturer and proceed with the scan. Anterior liver scans done with ^{131}I-rose bengal should be started at the lower edge of the liver, so that the gallbladder will not appear as a hot spot, since secretion from the liver is fairly rapid. Mark the dot or tap scan with the patient's name and the date, and note the instrument settings. On the anterior view, mark the xiphoid process (where the ribs meet the sternum), the rib margins, the lateral body margins and the umbilicus. Because of the shifts in the ability to concentrate labeled radiopharmaceuticals from liver to spleen to marrow, many centers have found it useful to record the count rate over the liver and spleen in the anterior view. This count can be obtained by moving the detector (with collimator on) over the liver and spleen, and noting the count rate produced on the count rate meter. Always ask a physician to palpate the abdomen to ascertain the location of the liver, spleen or other masses in the area. The marks representing location by palpation can be invaluable in interpretation of the scan. Transfer the information to the film after development.

For the lateral view, turn the patient so that he is lying on his left side, with right side up. Flexing the patient's knees will help maintain balance. In the lateral view, the collimator should be placed as close as possible to the skin so as to get a good view into the liver. Then proceed as in the anterior view. Obtain the same anatomic markings as for the anterior view.

The posterior view is the most desirable for visualizing the spleen.

The patient should be positioned lying prone on a stretcher, and the collimator face should be located so that the focal depth is about two inches below the skin. This position also provides a posterior view of the liver. The rib margins and spine should be marked on the dot or tap scan and transferred to the film after development.

As mentioned above, technetium sulfur colloid (TSC) is also removed from the bloodstream by the RE cells located in bone marrow. Thus, it is also possible to visualize the bone marrow of patients by injecting large amounts (up to 10 mCi) of ^{99m}Tc as TSC. Usually it is not possible to scan areas which overlie the liver and spleen. In some patients with far-advanced liver disease, the bone marrow may be the only region in which enough RE cells remain to provide the colloid removal function. In these patients, an attempt to obtain a liver scan will produce a bone marrow scan in that region.

The liver, spleen and bone marrow can also be visualized on the gamma-ray camera, but it is difficult to obtain on scintiphotos the anatomic information that is easily marked on rectilinear scans. Several technics have been proposed for obtaining such markings on liver scintiphotos, but none are completely satisfactory. Several liver-spleen scans and scintiphotos are shown in Figure 8-9. It can be seen that there are significant differences in the type of picture produced by the two instruments, with the rectilinear scanner providing a somewhat cleaner picture because of the focusing effect of the collimator. From 150,000 to 300,000 counts should be accumulated for each view obtained on the scintiphotos.

Fig. 8-9.—Rectilinear liver-spleen scans (*top row*) and scintiphotos (*bottom row*) obtained with gamma-ray camera. Note the effect of the focused collimator on the relative darkness of the organs in the anterior and posterior views. All scans and scintiphotos were obtained with ^{99m}Tc-sulfur colloid.

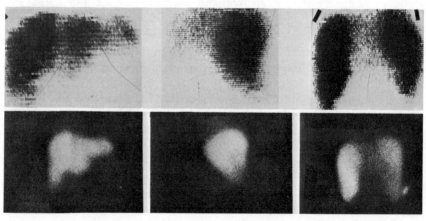

The pancreas is a common site for primary and metastatic cancer in the abdomen. Visualization of the pancreas by scanning is difficult at best, but can provide important diagnostic information. The scanning procedure depends on the physiology of the pancreas, which is an organ actively engaged in protein synthesis from amino acids. One of the essential amino acids, methionine, contains a sulfur atom that may be replaced by a selenium atom such as ^{75}Se (Fig. 8-10). Even with the substitution of ^{75}Se in the molecule, the pancreas and other organs treat the amino acid exactly as if it were methionine. Since ^{75}Se is radioactive with a half life of 127 days and produces gamma rays of 136 and 265 keV, areas of the body which are actively synthesizing protein from amino acids can be visualized by the rectilinear scanner or camera. Unfortunately, ^{75}Se-selenomethionine is also concentrated by the liver, an organ which may overlie the pancreas, so special scanning technics are required to observe the pancreas.

Approximately 200 μCi of ^{75}Se as selenomethionine is administered intravenously to adult patients, with smaller amounts for children. Some institutions have an elaborate preexamination procedure which may involve a fatty meal or drink. If such a test meal is required, ascertain that the patient has had the proper preparation before proceeding. Scanning with a rectilinear scanner or gamma-ray camera should begin within 30 minutes of injection. The patient should be in supine position on a stretcher, with the camera head placed below the rib margin and rotated slightly to look under the liver. Scintiphotos should be obtained about every 5 to 10 minutes with at least 50,000 counts collected for each photo. When using a rectilinear scanner, scanning should start below the liver and the scanner head should be tilted about 15 degrees; scanning should proceed upward toward the head. The instrument—either camera or scanner—should be peaked with a source of ^{75}Se. Care must be taken to peak on the 265-keV gamma ray, since the 136 keV photopeak of ^{75}Se is close to the 140-keV gamma ray of ^{99m}Tc which may also be present. The hot spot should be selected over the pancreas; the remaining instrument settings must be determined from the count rate and the manufacturer's recommendations. The patient's name, date and instrument settings are recorded on the dot or tap scan, as are the locations of rib margins, xiphoid, umbilicus and body margins; these are transferred

Fig. 8-10.—The chemical structure of methionine and ^{75}Se-selenomethionine.

$$CH_3 - S - CH_2 - CH_2 - \underset{\underset{COOH}{\diagdown}}{\overset{\overset{NH_2}{\diagup}}{C}}H \qquad CH_3 -^{75}Se - CH_2 - CH_2 - \underset{\underset{COOH}{\diagdown}}{\overset{\overset{NH_2}{\diagup}}{C}}H$$

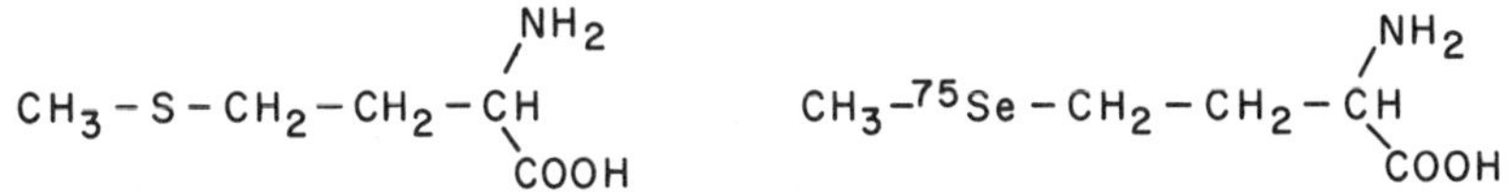

METHIONINE ^{75}Se-SELENOMETHIONINE

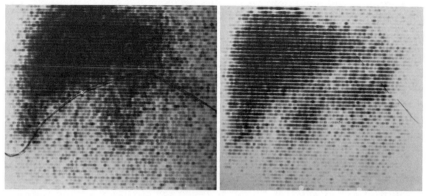

Fig. 8-11.—Pancreas scans obtained with ⁷⁵Se-selenomethionine. These scans are of above average quality; usually the pancreas is not so well separated from the liver. Both scans show normal organs.

to the film after development. Several good pancreas scans are shown in Figure 8-11; not all pancreas scans come out as well, however.

In order to better visualize the pancreas as an organ separate from the liver, many nuclear medicine centers obtain a liver scan with ⁹⁹ᵐTc-sulfur colloid immediately after the pancreas scan. If this is done, the ⁹⁹ᵐTc-sulfur colloid is administered intravenously to the patient before moving the stretcher or scanner. Scintiphotos or rectilinear scans are obtained with the gamma-ray camera or scanner in exactly the same position as the pancreas scan. The same anatomic information is marked on the liver scan or scintiphoto. This technic sometimes allows the pancreas to be visualized when the liver and pancreas are not clearly separated on the pancreas view alone.

PULMONARY FUNCTION STUDIES

The investigation of pulmonary function with radiopharmaceuticals has become one of the most important diagnostic examinations in nuclear medicine in recent years. Basically, there are two types of studies performed to evaluate lung function. The first study examines blood flow to the lungs and is called a perfusion examination. The second type is employed to evaluate the airflow into and out of the lungs and is called a ventilation, or wash-in–wash-out study. Both methods have become invaluable in observing regional function in the lungs; such observations are impossible with traditional pulmonary evaluation technics.

Perfusion function of the lungs can be evaluated by the intravenous injection of particles of human serum albumin (HSA) tagged with ¹³¹I or ⁹⁹ᵐTc. The HSA is first labeled with the radionuclide, then treated (usually by heating) to produce particles in the size range of 30 to 100 μ (3 × 10^{-3} to 10^{-2} cm.); the material is then called macroaggregated albumin (MAA). The particles, when injected into the venous circulation, travel to the heart and are pumped out to the lungs, where they are trapped in the capillary and precapillary vessels. Thus, perfusion scanning with MAA utilizes a physical or mechanical trapping to lodge the tagged particles in the lungs. There will be no blood flow, and thus no tagged particles in those areas of the lung in which perfusion has been compromised by a clot (embolism) or other pathologic condition. The particles themselves are uniformly distributed in the lungs, but approximately 1% of the blood flow through the lungs is cut off by the particles themselves.

Until 1971, only ^{131}I-labeled MAA was available for perfusion lung scans. Recently, ^{99m}Tc-MAA became commercially available. It will probably replace the ^{131}I-MAA because of a number of advantages it offers including reduced scanning time (more ^{99m}Tc can be used), lower internal radiation dose (because of the shorter half-life of ^{99m}Tc), and absence of secondary uptake (^{131}I may be taken up by the thyroid gland after the ^{131}I-MAA particles leave the lung and the ^{131}I is split off the albumin). As mentioned above, both agents are administered intravenously; the amount injected depends on the agent used. The usual adult dose is 250 μCi of ^{131}I-MAA or up to 5 mCi of ^{99m}Tc-MAA; these amounts should be scaled down for smaller patients.

For pulmonary studies, it is absolutely necessary that the patient be lying down as flat as possible when the radiopharmaceutical is injected. This is the only nuclear medicine procedure that requires a specific position during the time of injection. The reason that the patient must be flat is that blood flow and flow of the particles to various regions of the lungs are affected by position. In the normal patient lying flat, blood is nearly uniformly distributed throughout the lungs. A number of disease conditions (and patient positions) can produce changes in blood flow and particle distribution which would show up on the scan and affect the diagnosis. The absolutely supine position may be quite difficult for many patients who are in respiratory distress, but the time from injection of the labeled particle to their lodging in the lungs is only a few seconds. The patient may then be returned to a position in which he is more comfortable.

The lungs may be visualized on either a rectilinear scanner or gamma-ray camera. For the scanner, a dual-probe system has proved to be a considerable time saver; anterior and posterior views may be obtained at the same time, with one detector looking down at the patient's chest and the other looking up at the back. The dual-probe system is really two independent scanners with independent controls. Only the two collimated detectors move synchronously, so that the upper and lower probes must each be peaked for the isotope being used and the controls for each must be set for the correct speed, count rate, *etc*. The patient should be in supine position on a stretcher between the probes. Special stretchers are available that do not absorb large numbers of gamma rays leaving the patient in the direction of the lower probe. The patient should be scanned from the shoulders to below the rib margins. A glance at the dot or tap scan will indicate whether both lung fields are completely in the scan. The dot or tap scan should be marked with the patient's name, the instrument settings, and the anatomic locations of the sternal notch and xiphoid.

It has been shown that lateral views of the lungs obtained on rectilinear scanners are not representative of the distribution of the labeled particles in the lungs, apparently because the lungs shift position within the thoracic cavity when the patient is lying on his side.

The gamma-ray camera may also be used to obtain lung perfusion scintiphotos. The proper collimator must be selected, depending on the isotope used. Diverging collimators which are designed for optimum performance at about 400 keV are available from camera manufacturers. These collimators may be used with either ^{99m}Tc- or ^{131}I-MAA and have the advantage that both lungs may be visualized at the same time; however, this convenience is purchased at the cost of some loss in resolution and a reduced image size. Straight-hole collimators are usually not of sufficient size to visualize both lungs at the same time in an adult. If ^{131}I-MAA is used and only straight-hole collimators are available, a high-energy collimator is required. The low-energy collimator is acceptable for ^{99m}Tc-MAA studies. The gamma-ray camera also has a number of advantages for perfusion lung studies. Patients in severe respiratory distress may be examined sitting up and the scintiphoto usually is obtained in a shorter period than the scan. The mobility of the gamma-ray camera head allows oblique scintiphotos to be obtained with no patient discomfort.

Posterior and anterior views are obtained with the patient's back and chest, respectively, parallel to the face of the collimator. For ^{131}I-MAA, about 50,000 counts should be obtained to produce an adequate scintiphoto; the higher count rate produced by the larger quantities of ^{99m}Tc can be utilized to obtain at least 200,000 counts and thus provide a better scintiphoto for diagnostic purposes. Oblique views of both lungs should also be acquired to complete the study. These can be obtained by rotating the camera head to an angle of about 45 degrees, keeping the face of the collimator parallel to the patient's chest or back (Fig. 8-12).

These views provide visualization of peripheral lung areas that are not observed on the anterior or posterior views. A marker containing 10 to 20 μCi of ^{133}Ba ($t_{1/2}$ = 7.2 years, with a gamma ray at 363 keV) may be used to identify one side of the body on ^{131}I-MAA lung perfusion studies, and a ^{144}Ce or ^{57}Co marker can be employed for ^{99m}Tc-MAA scintiphotos.

Perfusion lung studies may also be obtained with a radioactive gas, xenon-133, dissolved in normal saline solution. The gas solution may be purchased from radiopharmaceutical manufacturers in sterile, pyrogen-free form. The ^{133}Xe solution is administered intravenously, travels through the right side of the heart, and is released into the lungs across the alveolar membrane. Approximately 95% of the ^{133}Xe in the blood is released in a single passage through the lungs. The ^{133}Xe is then exhaled as the patient breathes out. A gamma-ray camera is necessary to perform the study because the ^{133}Xe does not remain in the lungs long enough for rectilinear scanning. As with MAA studies, areas of the lung with compromised blood flow show up on the scintiphoto as regions with no radioactivity. An additional study is usually performed with ^{133}Xe in saline in a perfusion examination: sequential pictures are taken while the ^{133}Xe is removed from the lungs by exhalation. These later pictures provide valuable information about regional lung function in those areas where gas exchange is not occurring and where the ^{133}Xe tends to be retained and shows up as hot spots long after the radioactive gas has left other regions of the lung. This part of the examination is called a washout study.

Fig. 8-12.—Anterior and posterior oblique lung scintiphotos, with proper patient-camera position indicated.

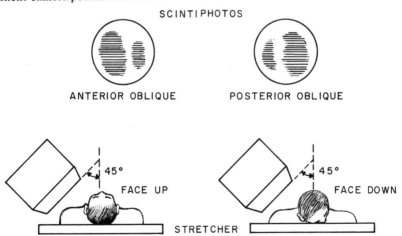

The radioactive gas ^{133}Xe has a half life of 5.3 days and its decay produces a gamma ray of 81 kev. In order to minimize radiation exposure to personnel, the patient undergoing an examination with ^{133}Xe should breathe directly into a system designed to trap or hold the radioactive gas. Several commercial systems are available for this purpose, but a simple system can be constructed using a Douglas bag, which is a large inflatable balloon, and asking the patient to exhale directly into the bag.

A similar study may be performed by administering ^{133}Xe as a gas with the air breathed by the patient. The examination is often called a wash-in – wash-out study, in that ^{133}Xe is inhaled until an equilibrium concentration in the lungs is attained; then the patient is allowed to breathe room air to provide the wash-out phase of the study. Once again, a gamma-ray camera is required because the ^{133}Xe does not remain in the lungs long enough to permit a scan. The ^{133}Xe gas is available from a number of sources and equipment for administering the gas to the patient is also commercially available. A system for trapping or holding the ^{133}Xe should be used for the gas studies.

With both intravenous administration of ^{133}Xe in solution and inhalation of ^{133}Xe gas, the patient is positioned with either his back or chest parallel to the face of the diverging collimator, which is used so that both lungs may be visualized. The patient should be lying flat, if possible, although this is not a strict requirement if a wash-in – wash-out study is being done. The gamma-ray camera should be peaked with a source of ^{133}Xe before starting. If a recording system (either magnetic tape or computer-coupled system) is available, it should be placed in operation in stand-by condition, ready to record data at the start of the examination.

For the perfusion wash-out study (intravenous injection of ^{133}Xe in solution), the recording system should be started at the time of injection. Dynamic scintiphotos can be obtained by exposing several Polaroid films (or 35- or 70-mm. camera film) for 5 to 10 seconds during the study. The first scintiphoto (0-5 seconds) will show entrance of the ^{133}Xe into the heart and lungs. The second (5-10 seconds) will show perfusion of the lungs. Later films will show the washing out of ^{133}Xe from the various regions. A recording system is invaluable, since it can be played back any number of times to provide more information.

When the ^{133}Xe is administered by inhalation, the film-exposure times should be lengthened to about 10 seconds and the recording system should be used if available. The wash-in part of this study takes longer than the perfusion examination because it takes longer to reach an equilibrium between inspired air and the added ^{133}Xe gas. The second part (wash-out) is exactly the same as the perfusion wash-out study. A typical

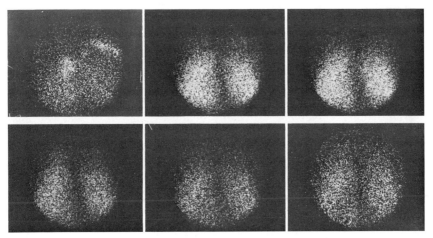

Fig. 8-13. — Perfusion and wash-out study obtained with ^{133}Xe and a gamma-ray camera fitted with a diverging collimator. The patient reached equilibrium, according to the spirometer, in about 30 seconds; this was followed by the wash-out phase.

perfusion ventilation study is shown in Figure 8-13. The marker button indicating the right side contained about 10 μCi of ^{144}Ce, which also has a gamma ray at 81 keV, in addition to the gamma ray at 136 keV, which makes ^{144}Ce useful as a marker on ^{99m}Tc scans.

RENAL STUDIES

The kidney performs a number of excretory functions for the body and the excretory function is utilized in nuclear medicine to obtain kidney scans and to evaluate the working of the kidneys. The kidneys perform their excretory job at two distinct levels: glomerular filtration and tubular filtration. The interested reader may find it helpful to study the physiology of the kidney in greater detail than can be included here. A number of radiopharmaceuticals are available that are removed from the blood by glomerular filtration; the radioactive atoms attached to the agents include ^{51}Cr, ^{99m}Tc, ^{131}I, ^{169}Yb, ^{197}Hg, and ^{203}Hg. Still other agents are removed from the bloodstream and become trapped in the kidneys; these materials are not usually desirable because the radiation dose to the kidneys can be very high unless the half life of the isotope is very short. The radiopharmaceuticals that are used for kidney studies and some of their important characteristics are listed in Table 8-3.

Kidney studies are becoming more numerous in nuclear medicine once again, after declining in popularity. Initially, there was great enthusiasm for a functional study in which ^{131}I-hippuran was administered intravenously and the removal, concentration, and excretion of the material was monitored with two scintillation detectors, one over each kidney. The count rate over each kidney was measured as a function of time, and many diagnostic inferences were drawn from the curve shapes. It turned out that the curves were not as specific as was first claimed, and kidney studies fell into some disrepute. With the availability of better kidney radiopharmaceuticals and the gamma-ray camera, renal studies are enjoying a comeback, especially in the evaluation of kidney transplants.

Renal scanning and functional studies are invaluable for those patients who are allergic to the iodine which is present in x-ray contrast agents and for patients who are in partial renal failure. The small amounts (by weight) of radioactive materials given for the nuclear medicine study will

TABLE 8-3.—SOME RADIOPHARMACEUTICALS USED FOR KIDNEY STUDIES

RADIOPHARMACEUTICAL	AMOUNT ADMINISTERED (ADULTS)	RADIONUCLIDE HALF LIFE	CHARACTERISTIC GAMMA RAYS	REMARKS
^{99m}Tc-DTPA*	2-5 mCi	6.0 hours	140 keV	Cleared by glomerular filtration and excreted. Good agent for function studies.
^{99m}Tc-DTPA (Squibb)*	2-5 mCi	6.0 hours	140 keV	Partially cleared by glomerular filtration, but not completely excreted. Good agent for kidney scans.
^{131}I-Hippuran	100-300 μCi	8.0 days	364 keV	Cleared by glomerular filtration. Good agent for function studies.
^{51}Cr EDTA†	100-300 μCi	27.8 days	320 keV	Cleared by glomerular filtration. Good agent for function studies.
^{197}Hg-Chlormerodrin	100-200 μCi	65 hours	77 keV	Concentrated in renal tubules. Not excreted. High radiation exposure to kidneys.

*DTPA is diethylenetriaminepentaacetic acid. This radiopharmaceutical is not the same as Squibb's DTPA, which contains iron and ascorbic acid and behaves quite differently from ^{99m}Tc-DTPA, as indicated above.
†EDTA is ethylenediaminetetraacetic acid.

not overburden an already taxed renal system. There is no iodine in most of the popular kidney radiopharmaceuticals, and the iodine in 300 μCi of ^{131}I is only about 2.4×10^{-9} Gm.

Almost any agent listed in Table 8-3 may be used for kidney scanning. Those radiopharmaceuticals cleared by glomerular filtration with excretion require that the scan be performed within 1 hour of the intravenous injection of the agent. The patient should be positioned prone on a stretcher under the scanner detector. The instrument should be peaked with the isotope used in the study (see Table 8-3 for gamma-ray energies). The hot spot should be selected over one of the kidneys, and machine settings should be on that count rate according to the manufacturer's directions. Mark the dot or tap scan with the patient's name and date, instrument settings, and rib and spine location. This information should be transferred to the film after development.

The gamma-ray camera can also be used effectively for kidney studies; both functional information as well as size and shape of the kidneys can be obtained. A recording device is very helpful for these studies. A diverging collimator should be used for all studies on normal adult patients, but a straight-hole collimator designed for the proper energy can be employed for children and kidney transplant examinations. The gamma-ray camera should be peaked for the isotope being used, and the recording equipment set to start when the radiopharmaceutical is injected. The usual patient will be positioned prone on a stretcher under the gamma-ray camera with the collimator face parallel to his back. The camera head should be centered over the patient's spine just above the

Fig. 8-14. – Renal study obtained with ^{99m}Tc-DTPA and a gamma-ray camera. The results of this study are normal; blood flow, concentration, and excretion are the same in both kidneys.

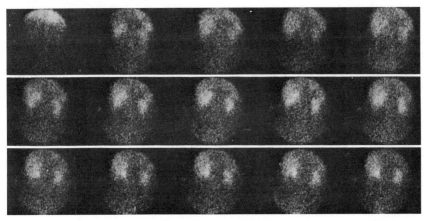

posterior rib margins. Kidneys are usually transplanted to the pelvic area, so transplant patients should be in supine position with the camera head over the transplant area; try to include the urinary bladder in the field of view, since urinary output from the transplanted kidney is an important parameter in the evaluation of transplant function.

The recording device should be started at the time the radiopharmaceutical is injected. Several scintiphotos should be obtained at 10- to 15-second intervals during the first minute after injection; these should show the blood supply to the kidneys and the initial concentration of the radiopharmaceutical. Several additional scintiphotos should then be taken at 5-minute intervals, up to about 30 minutes, to visualize the kidneys and their excretion of the labeled material. A marker with a gamma ray of the correct energy should be used to identify one side of the patient on the scintiphotos. A series of kidney scintiphotos obtained in a normal adult is shown in Figure 8-14.

BLOOD FLOW STUDIES

The blood supply to and through a number of organs is amenable to visualization by nuclear medicine instruments, particularly the gamma-ray camera. A number of radiopharmaceuticals have been used for these studies; the primary physical requirement for these agents is that they remain in the bloodstream at least for the period during which the study is performed. Human serum albumin (HSA) tagged with ^{99m}Tc or ^{131}I has been used for blood flow studies as well as ^{113m}In, which, when injected into the blood, forms a very stable complex with the plasma protein transferrin. The ^{113m}In has a half life of 104 minutes, emits a gamma ray of 394 keV, and is available from a ^{113}Sn-^{113m}In generator. The ^{113}Sn parent has a half life of 115 days. In these radiopharmaceuticals, the radionuclide remains permanently in the vascular system. Technetium-99m, as sodium pertechnetate, moves fairly rapidly from the blood into the extravascular space, so studies using this radiopharmaceutical must be performed within a few seconds of injection. Blood flow studies of the brain, lung, and kidneys have already been described in the sections on these organs. The only other principal organ system in which blood flow is currently investigated by nuclear medicine technics is the heart itself. As in other flow studies, a recording-playback system is required in order to get the most out of the study. Usually, 10 to 20 mCi of ^{99m}Tc is injected intravenously. The camera is located over the chest of the supine patient at an angle of about 45 degrees, similar to the position shown in Figure 8-12. The left oblique position provides a separation of both ventricles of the heart, whereas the right oblique position is very good for visualizing the left atrium. The recording system should be turned on at the moment of the injection and data should be recorded for 30 to 60 seconds. A cardiac study performed on a normal patient in the left oblique position is shown in Figure 8-15. The radioactive label can be seen flowing with the blood into the right atrium and ventricle, out the pulmonary artery to the lungs, back into the left ventricle, then out the aorta into the body. The study may be evaluated by selecting areas of interest in various parts of the heart and/or lung, and obtaining the count rate in each region selected. Basic physiologic information, especially the time required for blood to traverse from one region to the next, and the visualization of major cardiac defects can be obtained from such studies.

In addition to blood flow into and through an organ system, the radio-pharmaceuticals mentioned above (with the exception of ^{99m}Tc-sodium pertechnetate) have also been employed to establish the vascularity of lesions discovered in liver, lung, and brain scans. These studies may be performed with a rectilinear scanner or gamma-ray camera, since the changes in the concentration of radiopharmaceuticals are not so important here.

Another important study done with radiopharmaceuticals which stay in the blood is an examination designed to evaluate pericardial effusion. The pericardium is the tough sac which surrounds the heart; in certain diseases, fluid accumulates in the sac. On a chest x-ray, the heart appears enlarged, but it is usually not possible to differentiate between en-

Fig. 8-15.—Cardiac study performed in the left anterior oblique position using a gamma-ray camera and ^{99m}Tc as sodium pertechnetate.

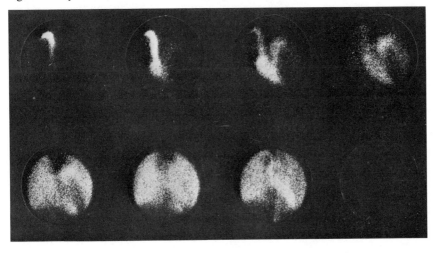

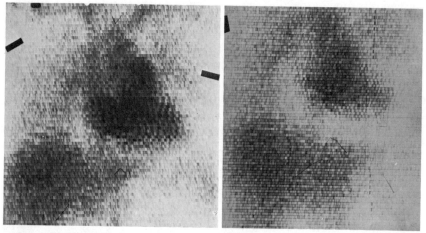

Fig. 8-16.—Rectilinear scans of the cardiac region. The radiopharmaceutical used was ^{113m}In. The scan on the left is of a normal patient, whereas the scan on the right shows a pericardial effusion (note the absence of the radiopharmaceutical in the region around the heart).

largement of the heart itself and pericardial effusion. Radiopharmaceuticals which remain in the blood will, of course, remain only in the heart and its circulatory system. Thus a scan or scintiphoto of the cardiac region will show whether the apparent enlargement of the heart results from an increase in the size of the heart or from pericardial effusion. Normal and abnormal pericardial scans are shown in Figure 8-16; the region around the heart in the latter scan is devoid of activity, indicating an effusion.

BONE STUDIES

The skeleton is one of the most troublesome systems for nuclear medicine examinations. Several common types of cancer, especially mammary cancer in women and prostatic cancer in men, can metastasize to bone. Patients with cancer of either the breast or prostate present formidable diagnostic problems in evaluating the spread of disease to the skeleton. One problem has been that at least 50% of the bone mineral must have been destroyed before such destruction is apparent in a radiograph. Bone scanning can provide information regarding skeletal metastases at a much earlier stage, but the technical problems of obtaining adequate bone scans are still great.

The bone mineral consists of a crystalline matrix of the compound known as hydroxyapatite which contains calcium, phosphate and hydroxyl ions. Most bone scanning agents have been developed by attempting to substitute a radioactive, gamma ray-emitting isotope of an element that is similar to the components of the bone mineral. Thus, ^{85}Sr and ^{87m}Sr are administered and are incorporated into the bone because strontium behaves chemically like calcium (see Chapter 2). In much the same way ^{18}F has been used for bone scanning; here the fluorine ions (F$^-$) take the place of hydroxyl ions (OH$^-$) in the bone. It is fair to say that the development of bone-scanning agents has been one of the most intensive areas of radiopharmaceutical research in the late 1960s and early 1970s. This work has produced a number of agents which have been reported to be effective bone-seeking materials. The most promising radiopharmaceutical reported has been technetium polyphosphate, which employs ^{99m}Tc and has shown exceptional properties as a bone-scanning agent.

The most commonly used bone-scanning radiopharmaceuticals and some of their important characteristics are listed in Table 8-4. The list is by no means complete, and further developments may make all of these agents obsolete. One of the major problems in designing a bone-scanning agent is the relatively slow rate of uptake of most materials in the bone; this means the half life of the tagging radionuclide must be long enough for the material to be cleared from the bloodstream and taken up by the bone, yet not so long as to produce an excessive radiation dose to the patient. Excretion via the kidneys and large intestine has been a continuing problem for the strontium and barium isotopes, since the pelvic region is an area of great interest in diagnosis.

All radiopharmaceuticals for bone scanning are administered intravenously in the amounts shown in Table 8-4. The use of ^{85}Sr is restricted by the United States Atomic Energy Commission to those patients with demonstrated cancer. With ^{85}Sr, scanning is performed 1 to 7 days after injection, but before scanning, the bowel must be thoroughly cleansed by providing the patient with a laxative and having him take an enema on the day of the scan. The shorter-lived radiopharmaceuticals (^{87m}Sr and ^{18}F) require that the scan be obtained between 1 and 3 hours after injection, and the patient is requested to void before the scan to eliminate the radioactivity accumulated in the urinary bladder. ^{99m}Tc-polyphosphate requires scanning within 4 to 8 hours post injection.

Both ^{18}F and ^{85}Sr require a rectilinear scanner for bone visualization because of the high energy of the gamma rays of these radionuclides. A scanner may also be preferred for the other radiopharmaceuticals because more of the patient can be visualized in a single view. At least one scanner manufacturer offers a "minification" option which provides a 5-

TABLE 8-4. — RADIOPHARMACEUTICALS COMMONLY USED FOR BONE SCANS

RADIOPHARMACEUTICAL	ADULT DOSE	RADIONUCLIDE HALF LIFE	CHARACTERISTIC GAMMA RAYS	REMARKS
^{85}Sr* (strontium nitrate)	100 μCi	65 days	513 keV	High radiation dose. Partially excreted in large intestine. Gamma-ray energy too high for gamma-ray camera.
^{87m}Sr (strontium nitrate)	1,000-2,000 μCi	2.80 hours	388 keV	Blood levels remain high during first hours. Early excretion in urine. Generator produced.
^{18}F (sodium fluoride)	1,000-2,000 μCi	1.87 hours	511 keV	Positron emitter. Accelerator produced. Excreted in urine. Gamma energy too high for gamma-ray camera.
^{131}Ba (barium chloride)	400-600 μCi	11.6 days	122 keV 214 keV 372 keV	Lower radiation dose than ^{85}Sr. Requires enriched ^{130}Ba.
^{99m}Tc (technetium polyphosphate)	10,000-15,000 μCi	6.0 hours	140 keV	Good localization in bone. Scanning done 4-6 hours after injection. Gamma-ray camera can be used.

*Use restricted by the United States Atomic Energy Commission to patients with proved cancer.

to-1 reduction in the size of the final scan. This option allows whole-body scans of patients to be obtained in less than an hour and is a distinct improvement in terms of patient comfort.

Be certain that the scanning instrument is peaked for the radionuclide administered to the patient. For ^{85}Sr, the "cold-spot" technic can produce fairly good bone scans. In contrast to the normal setting of the light-source voltage over a hot spot, the cold-spot technic consists of determining at what light-source voltage the film is minimally exposed at

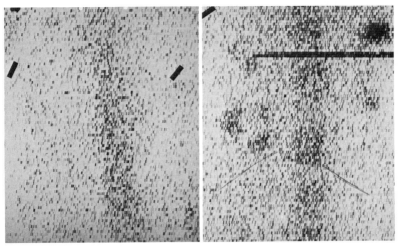

Fig. 8-17. — Bone scans obtained with ⁸⁵Sr. The left scan shows normal findings (negative for disease); the right scan shows abnormal uptake. Note the lack of high definition in both scans and the importance of symmetry in evaluating bone uptake.

a low-range differential setting (30 to 50). This voltage should be used when the detector is over normal bone; areas of increased uptake will then appear significantly darker than the normal areas. Use both probes if a dual-head scanner is available. The minimum bone scan consists of anterior and posterior views of the entire trunk of the patient's body, from neck to pelvis. Other regions (legs, arms, head) are not so frequently involved in metastatic disease, but may be sites of primary cancer. These areas would be included in a scan only on request by the referring physician. The dot or tap scan should be marked with the patient's name, the date, instrument settings, and anatomic markings (sternal notch, rib margins, pelvic brim, spine, pubic bone, and lateral body margins). The patient's right or left side must be clearly identified, since the interpretation of bone scans depends to a great extent on the amount of right-left symmetry observed on the scans. Two bone scans are shown in Figure 8-17. These were obtained on a 5-inch rectilinear scanner without minification, although photographic reproduction accomplishes essentially the same thing. The great improvement in bone scanning brought about by the use of ⁹⁹ᵐTc-polyphosphate can be seen in Figure 8-18. The definition in the scintiphotos is good enough to be able to distinguish ribs and vertebral bodies. Pathologic conditions show up as hot spots — areas that have accumulated more activity than normal bone.

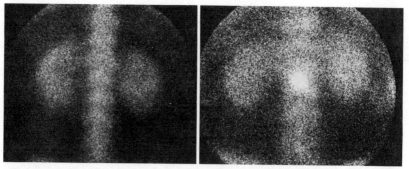

Fig. 8-18.—Bone scintiphotos obtained with ^{99m}Tc-polyphosphate. These scintiphotos were obtained 4 hours after injection of the material. The scinti-photo on the left shows a normal uptake in the skeletal system; the right scinti-photo shows metastatic involvement in the lumbar spine. Note the uptake of the radioactivity in the kidneys in both scintiphotos.

MISCELLANEOUS SCANNING AND SCINTIGRAPHY IN NUCLEAR MEDICINE

The scanning and gamma-ray procedures mentioned above cover more than 95% of the studies performed in nuclear medicine clinics at the present time. A number of diagnostic examinations may be per-formed with ^{75}Se-selenomethionine, which was mentioned earlier as a pancreas-visualizing agent. These procedures are based on the fact that ^{75}Se-selenomethionine is incorporated into protein and thus would be concentrated in any region in which active protein synthesis is occur-ring, particularly in rapidly growing tumors. A scan or scintiphoto might then be obtained at any area in which a tumor is suspected. Methionine has also been employed for visualization of the parathyroid glands, which are embedded in the thyroid gland. In this case, uptake of ^{75}Se-selenomethionine by the thyroid gland itself must be blocked by prior administration of the thyroid hormone triiodothyronine (T_3).

In a similar manner, any radiopharmaceutical which remains in the bloodstream (^{113m}In, ^{99m}Tc-human serum albumin) can be employed for visualizing areas which may have a rich blood supply. Both of these agents have been used for placental scanning in the diagnosis of placenta previa and in the examination of highly vascular tumors.

As the discussions in previous sections have indicated, the technician must be aware of the radioisotope being used in the study and the areas in which it is likely to be concentrated. Anatomic information should be marked on the dot or tap scan for localizing the area of the scan.

In Vitro Studies

In addition to the organ visualization procedures done in nuclear medicine, a number of other patient studies have grown up around the use of radionuclides in medicine. Although in vitro studies literally imply work performed in a test tube without the patient's presence, but using samples of blood, urine, or feces from the patient, several important nuclear medicine studies require the administration of radioactive materials to the patient. In other tests, the patient does not receive any radioactive material, but radionuclides are used to perform the test. In all the in vitro tests described here, no distinction is made between these types of tests; the only requirement is that radioactivity in a sample be counted rather than radioactivity in a patient.

The Schilling Test

The Schilling test measures the metabolism of vitamin B_{12}. The absorption of this important vitamin requires the presence of a compound called intrinsic factor, which is produced or activated in the gastric mucosa. Although other disease states may prevent absorption, the most common cause of malabsorption is the lack of intrinsic factor found associated with pernicious anemia. Vitamin B_{12} contains cobalt, and the normal cobalt may be replaced with radioactive cobalt—usually ^{57}Co or ^{60}Co. The decay characteristics of these isotopes are summarized in Table 8-5. The test is relatively simple to perform and provides valuable diagnostic information. After overnight fasting, the patient receives an oral dose of vitamin B_{12} (1.0 μg) tagged with 0.5 μCi of ^{57}Co or ^{60}Co. The tagged vitamin is available in capsules from a number of radiopharmaceutical manufacturers. Two hours after the patient receives the tagged capsule of vitamin B_{12}, 1,000 μg of vitamin B_{12} is injected intra-

TABLE 8-5.—CHARACTERISTICS OF COBALT ISOTOPES USED FOR SCHILLING TESTS

ISOTOPE	HALF LIFE	GAMMA RAYS	REMARKS
^{57}Co	270 days	122 keV	Isotope of choice. Gamma-ray energy close to ^{99m}Tc (140 keV).
^{60}Co	5.3 years	1.17 MeV 1.33 MeV	High-energy gamma rays. May be useful if patient has had other nuclear medicine studies.

muscularly. This injection saturates the B_{12} binding sites in the body, so the tagged B_{12} is excreted in the urine rather than retained in the body. The patient's urine is collected for 24 hours and the volume measured. A small volume of urine (10 to 20 ml) is removed and the radioactivity therein is counted; the radioactivity in a standard containing a known amount of ^{57}Co (or ^{60}Co, if this isotope is used) is also counted. The standard may be prepared by dissolving a 0.5 μCi capsule in 1,000 milliliters of water and removing a 10.0 ml. sample for counting. The total activity excreted in the urine in 24 hours is calculated by comparing the urine count with the standard count. An equation for the calculation of the excretion is

$$\% \text{Excretion} = \frac{C_S \times V_E \times V_{STD} \times 100}{C_{STD} \times V \times V_S} \qquad (8\text{-}2)$$

in which C_S is the net count rate of the urine sample in counts per minute,

V_S is the volume of the urine sample counted in milliliters,

V_E is the total urine volume excreted in milliliters,

C_{STD} is the net count rate of the standard in counts per minute,

V_{STD} is the volume of the standard taken for counting in milliliters, and

V is the initial volume to which the standard was made up.

Normal values for the Schilling test are in the range of 10 to 40%. If the excretion is below 10%, the test should be repeated with intrinsic factor given orally at the same time as the vitamin B_{12}. The remainder of the test is exactly the same as the test without intrinsic factor. If the excretion is still below 10%, pernicious anemia can usually be ruled out.

BLOOD VOLUME DETERMINATION

The volume of blood in the body may be determined by the intravenous injection of a known amount of labeled material which remains in the bloodstream. Radiopharmaceuticals such as ^{51}Cr-labeled red blood cells (a small amount of the patient's own blood is withdrawn, labeled and reinjected), or ^{131}I- or ^{99m}Tc-human serum albumin may be used. A small measured amount (5 to 10 μCi) of the radiopharmaceutical is injected and allowed to circulate for 5 to 10 minutes. Then a blood sample is withdrawn and the radioactivity in a known volume (1.0 or 2.0 ml.) is counted. The blood should be stored in a tube containing heparin or other anticlotting agents; otherwise the blood will form a clot and erroneous results will ensue. A standard is prepared by diluting the same measured amount of the same radiopharmaceutical (5 to 10 μCi) to a known volume — 1,000 ml. The radioactivity in a known volume of the standard is then counted. The blood volume is given by the following equation:

$$\text{Blood Volume (ml.)} = \frac{C_{STD} \times V_B \times V}{C_B \times V_{STD}} \tag{8-3}$$

in which C_{STD} is the net count rate of the standard in counts per minute, V_B is the volume of blood counted in milliliters, V is the volume to which the standard was diluted in milliliters, C_B is the net count rate of the blood in counts per minute, and V_{STD} is the volume of the diluted standard counted in milliliters.

Remember that *exactly* the same amount of radiopharmaceutical must be injected into the patient as is used to prepare the solution from which the standard volume is diluted. The blood volume is usually reported in terms of the weight of the patient—milliliters per kilogram of body weight—so the value provided by equation 8-3 must be divided by the patient's weight in kilograms. Normal values are in the range of about 70 to 90 ml./kg.

RED CELL SURVIVAL

The rate of disappearance of red blood cells from the blood is measured indirectly in this test. Red blood cells are taken from a patient, tagged with ^{51}Cr and reinjected. Thereafter, blood samples are obtained every 2 to 4 days for 2 to 4 weeks. The tagging of red blood cells with ^{51}Cr involves removing about 25 ml. of whole blood from the patient and placing it in a sealed vial containing acid citrate dextrose (ACD) solution. About 50 μCi of ^{51}Cr-sodium chromate is added to this mixture, which is then incubated for about 15 minutes to label the red cells. The mixture is then treated with ascorbic acid to stop further labeling. The tagged red cells are washed to remove unbound ^{51}Cr, resuspended in saline solution, and reinjected into the patient. After 15 to 20 minutes of equilibration, a blood sample is withdrawn and saved as a standard or 100% value. This sample and others obtained later should be stored in tubes containing an anticlotting agent. After all the samples have been collected, accurately measured volumes of each are obtained and the radioactivity in each is counted. The counting rate of each sample is expressed as a percentage of the initial or 100% sample. The percentage is plotted on the log scale of semilog graph paper as a function of time. The data points are then connected by a straight line from which the half time is determined (the test results are handled in much the same way as the half life of a radionuclide is measured—see Chap. 5). The normal value for ^{51}Cr-tagged red cell survival is about 30 days.

T_3-RESIN UPTAKE AND T_4 TESTS

The T_3-resin uptake test and T_4 assay are two thyroid function tests that are performed in vitro. Kits for performing both tests are available from a number of radiopharmaceutical manufacturers, and the instructions must be followed exactly to obtain accurate results.

The T_3 uptake test measures the degree of saturation of thyroxine-binding globulins (TBG) in the blood plasma of the patient. The test is performed by adding ^{125}I- or ^{131}I-labeled triiodothyronine (T_3) to a sample of the patient's plasma. A material having secondary T_3 binding sites (ion-exchange resin or red blood cells) is also present in the vial or tube. After incubation for about an hour, the radioactivity of the contents of the vial is counted; then the plasma and the secondary binding site material are separated and their radioactivity is counted. The patient sample and a standard (pooled) plasma sample are done at the same time. The results may be reported as per cent uptake in the secondary binding material (normal range 30 ± 5%, but this may vary) or as a percentage of the T_3 uptake of the standard plasma (100 ± 10% is usually considered normal, but each laboratory should establish a normal range of values). Instructions provided with commercial kits also provide information on ranges for hypo-, eu-, and hyperthyroid patients, as well as important cautions regarding the effects of various drugs and medical conditions on the test results.

Since the T_3 uptake (and the uptake of radioactive iodine) may be affected by a large amount of iodine in the patient's system, producing clinically nonsensical results, an effort has been made to develop a test which is not affected by the amount of iodine in the patient. This has produced the so-called T_4 test, which measures the amount of circulating thyroxine (T_4) in the patient's plasma. There are a number of commercial kits available which can be used to perform the test. They are quite varied in their degree of complexity, and once again, the directions must be followed exactly to produce clinically useful results.

RADIOIMMUNOASSAY

A complete discussion of the methods and technics of radioimmunoassay will not be attempted in this book. Basically, the technic can be used to measure the extremely low concentrations of a number of hormones that are of great medical importance. The method, which was developed by Yalow and Berson around 1960, was first used to measure insulin levels in blood at levels of 10^{-6} to 10^{-9} gram per liter of blood. The principle of the radioimmunoassay procedure is indicated in Figure 8-19. Labeled hormone binds to a specific antibody to form a labeled antigen-antibody complex. However, the formation of labeled complex can be made competitive with the formation of unlabeled antigen-antibody

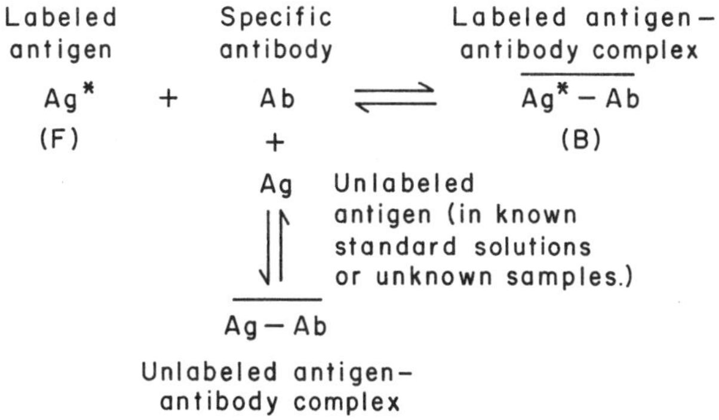

Labeled antigen	Specific antibody	Labeled antigen–antibody complex
Ag*	+ Ab ⇌	Ag* – Ab
(F)	+	(B)

Ag Unlabeled antigen (in known standard solutions or unknown samples.)

⇅

Ag – Ab

Unlabeled antigen–antibody complex

Fig. 8-19.—The basic reactions of radioimmunoassay.

complex by adding unlabeled antigen (obtained from a standard of the hormone under investigation or from the patient's blood). As a result of the competition, the ratio (B:F) of antibody bound (B) to free (F) hormone decreases as the concentration of the unlabeled hormone increases. The method simply requires a method for separating the antigen-antibody complex (labeled [*] and unlabeled) from the uncomplexed antigen.

The technic can be extended to nonhormone systems if the proper reactants can be obtained, as indicated in Figure 8-20. A specific reactant (R) is chosen which reacts only with the labeled substrate (S*) to form a S*-R complex. As in radioimmunoassay, the addition of unlabeled substrate (S) competes with S* to form the S-R complex, and the ratio (B:F) of bound (B) and free (F) labeled substrate decreases as the amount of unlabeled substrate added increases. Again, there must be a method for separating the complex from the unbound substrate. The principle has been applied to a number of hormones including insulin, human growth hormone, and thyroid and parathyroid hormones, as well

Fig. 8-20.—The extension of radioassay technic to nonhormone systems.

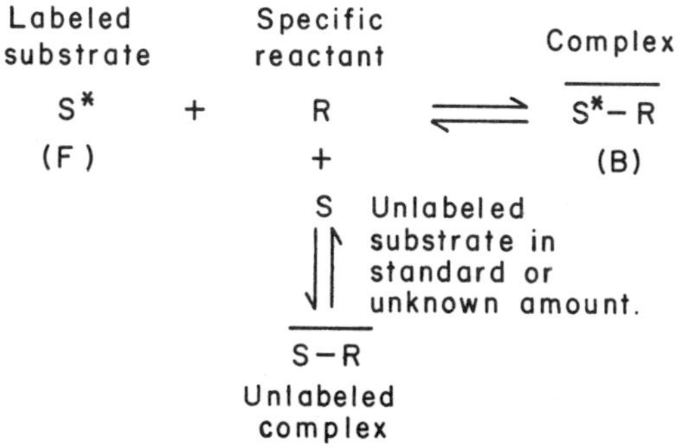

Labeled substrate	Specific reactant	Complex
S*	+ R ⇌	S* – R
(F)	+	(B)

S Unlabeled substrate in standard or unknown amount.

⇅

S – R

Unlabeled complex

as nonhormone systems such as vitamin B_{12}, folic acid, and digoxin. Several manufacturers have started manufacturing kits for radioimmunoassay in which everything is included but the counter. Most kits included a calibration curve in which the B:F ratio is plotted as a function of the concentration of the material being studied. As in all kit systems, the directions must be followed exactly to provide accurate results. It seems likely that the use of these kits will expand greatly, with more and more laboratories being set up to perform assays of these materials.

SUGGESTED READING

Blahd, W. H. (ed.): *Nuclear Medicine* (2d ed.; New York: McGraw-Hill Book Company, 1971).

Maynard, C. D.: *Clinical Nuclear Medicine* (Philadelphia: Lea and Febiger, 1969).

Silver, S.: *Radioactive Nuclides in Medicine and Biology: Medicine* (3d ed.; Philadelphia: Lea and Febiger, 1968).

Wagner, H. N., Jr. (ed.): *Principles of Nuclear Medicine* (Philadelphia: W. B. Saunders Co., 1968).

STUDY QUESTIONS

1. Define the terms sterility and freedom from pyrogens.
2. Ascertain the requirements for obtaining a license to use radiopharmaceuticals in your hospital.
3. What radioisotopes are used to study thyroid function?
4. Describe the different kind of information provided by the following thyroid tests: (a) thyroid uptake, (b) thyroid scan, and (c) T_3 and T_4 tests.
5. Explain how a thyroid uptake test is performed.
6. What is the basic principle behind brain scanning with radioactive isotopes?
7. How does a cerebrospinal fluid study differ from a brain scan? What radiopharmaceuticals are used for these two studies?
8. Compare and contrast brain scanning performed with a rectilinear scanner and a gamma-ray camera.
9. What premedication is required for brain scanning, and why is it used?
10. What radiopharmaceuticals may be used for liver scanning? Describe the physiologic process responsible for localization of each agent in the liver.
11. What other organs can be visualized with the various liver-scanning radiopharmaceuticals?
12. Describe the physiologic process responsible for localization of ^{75}Se-selenomethionine in the pancreas.
13. Compare and contrast pulmonary perfusion and ventilation studies performed with radiopharmaceuticals, including a discussion of the isotopes used and their mechanism of localization in the lungs.
14. What radiopharmaceuticals may be used for renal studies? Describe the mechanism of localization in the kidneys for each.
15. What is the main characteristic required of a radiopharmaceutical to be used for blood flow studies? What organ systems can be investigated with such agents?
16. Describe the radiopharmaceuticals used for bone scanning and the mechanism of localization of each agent.

CHAPTER 9

Health Physics

THE GREAT INCREASE in the number and kind of medical procedures utilizing ionizing radiation has had an enormous effect on almost everyone's sensitivity and awareness of the hazards associated with ionizing radiation. Although not all the answers have been provided for all the questions asked regarding the biologic effects of radiation, there is a great deal now known. The aim of this chapter is to provide the technologist with sufficient knowledge and understanding of the effects of ionizing radiation to be able to protect himself from the hazards and to provide reassuring information to the inquisitive patient.

Health Physics Units and Measurements

From the time of discovery of x-rays and nuclear radiation, there has been considerable confusion regarding units and their definition. Only a few well-accepted units will be introduced and defined here in order to eliminate confusion.

The basic unit of exposure is the roentgen (R). Note that this is an *exposure* unit, and says nothing at all about the amount of radiation *absorbed*. The official definition of 1.0 R is "that exposure of x- or gamma radiation such that the associated corpuscular emission per 0.001293 gram of air, produces in air, ions carrying one electrostatic unit of electricity of either sign." Briefly, this means that in 1.00 cc. of air at 0 C. and atmospheric pressure of 760 mm. of mercury (weight = 0.001293 gm.), 1.00 R of exposure will produce ions and electrons (corpuscular emissions). Since each of the singly charged ions and electrons carries a charge of 4.80×10^{-10} electrostatic units, this indicates that about 2×10^9 (two billion) ions and electrons are produced. Note that the definition says nothing about the time required to produce the roentgen exposure. The exposure measured on portable ionization chambers or calibrated Geiger counters is usually in R per minute or R per hour, so that the total exposure is the rate in R per unit time multiplied by the time of exposure. The definition may be applied to electromagnetic radiation up to 3 MeV only.

Obviously, if one is exposed to ionizing radiation, some of it will be absorbed by the various ways in which ionizing radiation interacts with matter. The unit of radiation absorbed dose is the *rad*, which is defined as the absorption of 100 ergs per gram of tissue. There is a definite relationship between radiation exposure in roentgens and radiation absorbed dose in rads. For most practical purposes, one roentgen of exposure will produce a radiation absorbed dose of one rad. To return to the definition of the rad, the absorbed dose is 100 ergs per gram of tissue. As mentioned in Chapter 3, the erg is a small amount of energy, but the usual measure of gamma-ray energy—the MeV—is much smaller, since one MeV = 1.6×10^{-6} erg. A quick calculation will show that the complete absorption of 6.25×10^7 (62.5 million) gamma rays of 1 MeV absorbed in a gram of tissue will produce a radiation absorbed dose of one rad. If the same number of 1-MeV gamma rays were absorbed in a tissue sample of 100 grams, the radiation absorbed dose would be 0.01 rad (1.0 rad per 100 grams).

Up to this point, the discussion has been limited to x- and gamma radiation. The roentgen is limited to this type of radiation, but the rad is not. There are other types of ionizing radiation, i.e., alpha and beta particles, conversion electrons, neutrons, *etc.* It has been determined that the more heavily ionizing particles (alpha and neutrons) are much more effective in producing biologic damage than x-rays, gamma rays and electrons. To provide for this difference, the concept of relative biologic effectiveness (RBE) has been introduced. The radiation absorbed dose in *rads* is multiplied by the RBE to give the equivalent radiation absorbed dose in *rems*. The RBE factors for fast neutrons and alpha particles are 10 and 20, respectively. The RBE for x-rays, gamma rays and electrons is one. Thus, if 6.25×10^7 alpha particles of 1.0 MeV energy are absorbed in one gram of tissue, the rad dose would be 1.0 rad, but the equivalent radiation absorbed dose would be 20 rems. An important point to recall in thinking about radiation absorbed dose is the fact that all particulate radiations (alpha, beta, conversion electrons) give up all their energy in a very short path length in tissue—within a fraction of a millimeter of the site of decay. Thus, the local radiation absorbed dose from particulate radiation will be much greater than from gamma or x-rays.

Background Radiation

Everyone is exposed to ionizing radiation which arises from a variety of sources in nature over which no one has control. This natural background of ionizing radiation can be divided into two types of sources, external and internal. The external background exposure comes from cosmic rays which originate in outer space and carry enormous amounts

TABLE 9-1.— AVERAGE RADIATION
ABSORBED DOSE IN REM/PERSON/YEAR IN
THE UNITED STATES CAUSED BY NATURAL
AND ARTIFICIAL SOURCES

SOURCE	WHOLE BODY DOSE rem/Person/Year
Cosmic rays	0.03
Natural radioactivity	0.05
Internal radionuclides	0.025
Total natural	0.1
Medical and dental x-rays	0.15–0.35
Occupational	0.005
Fallout	0.015–0.020
Total artificial	0.17–0.33
Total, all sources	0.3–0.4

of energy. Internal sources include the naturally occurring radioactive elements which are part of the human body. The most common sources of naturally occurring internal radiation exposure are ^{40}K and ^{14}C. The adult human body contains a total of about 150 grams of potassium, of which 0.012% is ^{40}K. This means that each adult contains about 0.018 gram of radioactive ^{40}K, which has a half-life of 1.3×10^9 years. Using equation 5-4, it is possible to calculate that this amount of ^{40}K is equal to 0.124 μCi, or 2.74×10^5 disintegrations per minute. This rate of decay goes on continuously for a lifetime and produces a constant radiation absorbed dose in everyone.

In addition to these naturally occurring sources of ionizing radiation, there are a number of artificial, man-made, radiation-exposure sources over which some control can be exercised. These sources include medical and dental x-rays, occupational exposure (radioisotopes, radium, x-ray technology), and "fallout" from nuclear weapons testing, nuclear reactor operations and nuclear reactor fuel fabrication and reprocessing. The average absorbed dose to the general population of the United States from all sources is summarized in Table 9-1. The average total radiation absorbed dose is approximately 0.35 rem.

Biologic Effects of Radiation

It has been demonstrated that the general population absorbs a fair amount of ionizing radiation each year. The questions that now arise concern the effects of this absorbed dose on the individual, and the effects of increased exposure on the person who absorbs much more than the average amount during the performance of his job. One of the important aspects of ionizing radiation is that there is a fairly wide range of response to a given amount of radiation absorbed dose, so that it is difficult to specify exactly what will occur after a given amount of radiation has been absorbed in a biologic system. For example, in man, a whole-body radiation absorbed dose of approximately 500 rads will be lethal to about 50% of the population.

The biologic effects of radiation can be divided into two classes, somatic and genetic damage. Somatic effects include the immediate and late results of exposure to radiation. Depression of white blood cell count (leukopenia), skin reddening (erythema), nausea, vomiting, loss of hair (epilation), and massive cell death are usually considered to be the immediate somatic effects of overexposure; tumor induction, sterility, leukemia, cataracts, and life shortening are some of the late effects. It is difficult to specify the radiation absorbed dose required to produce these effects because there is apparently a relationship between the rate of exposure and the biologic damage. A single whole-body dose of 500 rads would prove fatal to about half of the population, but if this absorbed dose were spread over 50 years, there would be no deaths attributable to immediate effects. Still, the incidence of late effects would probably produce a net shortening of life.

The estimation of radiation absorbed dose required to produce somatic effects is based on several different sources of information in which attempts have been made to correlate radiation absorbed dose with biologic damage. Some information has been obtained from occupational exposure records — mostly from a group of people who were involved in painting radium on watch dials. These dial painters habitually pointed their paint brushes with their lips and tongue, and in this way managed to acquire a body burden of radium. Also, in the 1920s and early 1930s, a large number of patients were treated for an amazing variety of diseases with a drink containing radium salts. Additional information has been obtained from a few accidental radiation overexposures at atomic energy facilities throughout the world.

Diagnostic and therapeutic radiologic procedures have been performed on patients for about 60 years, and relatively good information has been provided by these intentional exposures, at least for low-energy x- and gamma radiation. A third type of information has been produced as a result of many experiments on lower animals, mainly rats, mice, and the famous fruit fly. However, the extrapolation of the results of these experiments to human beings is risky business at best. A fourth source of knowledge about radiation effects has been the continuing exhaustive study of the survivors of the atomic bomb explosions at Hiroshima and

Nagasaki carried out by the Atomic Bomb Casualty Commission under the auspices of the United States Atomic Energy Commission.

The local absorption of a single dose of several hundred rads is apparently enough to cause skin reddening which will disappear within a few weeks. Chronic skin absorption of several hundred rads per year over a period of years may produce late effects such as dry skin which is subject to cracking and ulceration, and eventually, tumor production. Approximately 400 rads absorbed locally in the eye will produce cataract, although the time between exposure and cataract formation may be several years.

A number of animal experiments have shown a definite shortening of life span for chronically irradiated animals, and although there are no accurate statistical studies of life shortening in man resulting from chronic low exposure to radiation, there probably will ultimately prove to be a correlation between decreased life span and radiation absorbed dose.

One of the greatest dangers of ionizing radiation is to the unborn child, especially in the first 3 months of pregnancy. One estimate of the amount of absorbed dose sufficient to produce serious abnormalities in the fetus during this period is as low as 50 rads. The United States Atomic Energy Commission has recently promulgated a rule designed to minimize radiation exposure to occupational workers who are pregnant. The ruling is that during the full 9-month term of pregnancy, the radiation absorbed dose of the mother shall not exceed 0.500 rads.

In addition to these serious somatic effects, more and more interest in recent years has centered on the genetic effects of the absorption of ionizing radiation. Genetic defects can be caused by ionizing radiation through damage to the chromosomal material that makes up everyone's genetic heritage. This chromosomal damage may occur in the egg cell of the female or the sperm cell of a male. If either the egg or the sperm which unite to form an offspring carries a chromosomal defect, the offspring will be a mutant, a result of chromosomal mutation. Mutants are of two types, dominant and recessive. A dominant mutation will produce a mutant offspring from the joining of a normal sperm or egg with a mutant egg or sperm carrying a dominant mutation. A recessive trait will be expressed in the offspring only if both parent cells contain the mutant. Thus, a recessive mutation may be produced and not be expressed for a number of generations, although the potential for expression is always present. A dominant mutational defect may be so serious that the offspring may not survive even the first few hours of life, and the mutation will immediately die out. Thus, it is the increase in the number of recessive chromosomal defects that is the major concern. It is now apparent that the evolution of man proceeded slowly by such recessive mutations, and presumably this genetic evolution is continuing at the present time. It is a matter of conjecture as to what is the driving force behind evolutionary development, but apparently the natural background of ionizing radiation was one of the causes.

So the question of genetic damage must rest on the problem of how great a genetic change caused by man-made ionizing radiation can be considered acceptable. The problem is often discussed in terms of the radiation absorbed dose which would be required to double the number of mutations in the whole population. The doubling dose rests on the assumption that a state of equilibrium with regard to recessive traits exists in which some mutations are being eliminated with time as others are added, and the number of genetic defects carried by the population as a whole would be increased by a factor of two by the doubling dose. An analysis of the effects of the doubling dose is rather complex, but several extreme conditions can be easily understood. For dominant mutations, a single doubling dose to one generation will double the number of dominant traits in the next generation; however, this dominant trait would be diluted in succeeding generations. If the doubling dose were continued for many generations, equilibrium would be established at twice the initial mutation rate. For recessive traits, a single doubling dose would produce a very small change in the succeeding generation; for a permanently doubled dose, more than 50 generations would be required to increase the recessive mutation rate by 50%. These are extreme examples, of course, but they do provide order of magnitude estimates of what would occur. Note that this doubling dose would have to be applied to the whole population in order for these effects to be observed. If only a small portion of the population received the doubling dose, the effects would be extremely small, even after very many generations.

There is considerable difficulty in establishing the magnitude of the doubling dose; estimates vary from 25 to 150 rads, but generally accepted values are in the range of about 50 rads. The difficulties in establishing the doubling dose result from the fact that very little information is available on the genetic effects of ionizing radiation in human beings. Large numbers of experiments have been performed on the fruit fly and mice and rats, but extrapolation of the data to man is hazardous. One speculation regarding the genetic effects of ionizing radiation is that there is apparently no threshold. This means there is no radiation dose level below which there are no genetic effects. However, it is probably impossible to prove this speculation on a statistical basis, even with fruit flies, since the number of experimental animals which would have to be irradiated at the lowest dose rates to establish the existence of a threshold would be enormous. At the present time, we are left with the unhappy prospect that even the slightest increase in radiation exposure increases the risk of genetic damage.

Recommended Exposure Limits

The International Committee on Radiation Protection (ICRP) and, in the United States, the National Committee on Radiation Protection (NCRP) have established limits on the radiation absorbed dose for occupationally exposed persons (atomic energy plant employees, x-ray workers, nuclear medicine workers) and the general population. These limits are called the maximum permissible dose (MPD) limits. The MPD limits are based on exposures in rems, which is the rad dose multiplied by the RBE factor. The MPD limits vary with the organ or organ system being considered. The present MPD limit for the whole body, lens of the eye, or gonads is given by:

$$\text{MPD} = 5\,(N-18)\ \text{rem} \qquad (9\text{-}1)$$

in which N is the subject's age in years. This means that a person 18 years of age who undertakes an occupation for which there is a radiation exposure hazard may receive up to 5 rems per year. If occupational entry occurs after age 18, the initial annual exposure may exceed 5 rems, but may not exceed 12 rems per year. Note that occupational exposure should not start before age 18. The 5 rems per year limit averages out to slightly less than 0.1 rem (100 millirem) per week, but there are provisions in the rules which permit higher dose rates. For example, up to 3 rems may be accumulated in a 13-week quarter as long as the annual dose does not exceed 5 rems.

Since the hands, arms, legs and feet are much less sensitive than the organs mentioned above, the MPD limits for the hands, arms, legs and feet are considerably higher. Their annual MPD limit is 75 rems, rather than the 5 rems mentioned above. The same 13-week quarterly fluctuations (up to 45 rems per quarter, but not to exceed 75 rems per year) are permitted. In none of these MPD limits is nonoccupational exposure considered, so a film badge should not be worn during dental or medical x-ray procedures, nor when receiving radioisotopes for diagnostic or therapeutic purposes. The recommended MPD limits for exposure in the general population are one tenth of those for occupational exposure; however, there are no established limits for medical exposure from diagnostic or therapeutic x-rays or radioisotopes. The administered exposure dose is left to the judgment of the physician in charge, who is expected to be able to judge the risks of exposure against the possible benefits to be gained from the examination or treatment.

Personnel Monitoring

One of the prerequisites for obtaining a license to use radionuclides is the establishment of an adequate personnel monitoring system for the people who will be exposed to the radiations from the radioisotopes. In most institutions at the present time, personnel exposure monitoring is done by requiring all personnel to wear a film badge at all times during exposure to radiation.

A film badge consists of a piece of dental (no-screen) x-ray film enclosed in a light-tight envelope. A number of commercial firms provide a monthly film change and reading for each badge wearer. The film holder may be as simple as a clip to attach the film to the wearer's clothing, or complex in that a series of absorbers may be stacked in shingle fashion over the film in an attempt to estimate the energy and type of radiation exposure.

The film should be removed and read at monthly intervals; it should be read even more frequently when exposures may be higher than normal. During nonworking hours, the film should be stored away from sources of ionizing radiation. (An apparent overexposure of several technicians and physicians at Yale was solved when it was found that each night these people left their lab coats, with film badges attached, on a coat rack next to a particular wall. On the other side of the wall was a refrigerator containing the usual inventory of radiopharmaceuticals for a busy nuclear medicine section.)

The film is "read" by development under rigidly standardized conditions and the degree of film blackening is measured with an optical densitometer. The densitometer readings are compared to those of films exposed to known standard radiation doses. The lower limit of sensitivity is about 10 millirem; on a monthly basis, this is about 2.5% of the MPD limit.

In addition to the film badge for personnel monitoring, several institutions have initiated an exposure-measuring system based on thermoluminescent dosimetry (TLD). Certain chemical compounds such as lithium fluoride and calcium fluoride have a unique property which makes them very useful for monitoring radiation exposure. When these compounds absorb ionizing radiation at room temperature, the crystalline structure of the material is changed; in effect, the energy absorbed is stored in the form of these structural changes in the crystals. When the compounds are heated rapidly, the crystal structure returns to its initial state, and the stored energy is released in the form of visible light—thus the term thermoluminescence. The amount of light produced on heating is proportional to the amount of energy absorbed by the material. The crystalline compounds and instrument systems for measuring the light output are available from a number of manufacturers. The TLD system has a number of advantages over film dosimetry, including the ease with which the dosimeters can be read, and the fact that the dosimeter materials can be used again and again. In addition, the TLD materials have a much wider dose range—from 0.1 rad to more than 10,000 rads—and the relatively low atomic number of the lithium fluoride makes the material nearly equivalent to body tissue in absorption properties. It seems likely that TLD systems will ultimately replace the film badge dosimetry presently used in most institutions.

Personnel Protection

The personnel monitoring systems do not provide any protection from exposure to ionizing radiation. The hazards of exposure to ionizing radiation must be dealt with according to three principles: quantity of radioactive material, time of exposure, and distance from the source of radiation. The absorbed dose is directly proportional to the amount of radioactivity and the time of exposure, and inversely proportional to the square of the distance from source to absorber. The radiation absorbed dose may be sharply reduced by shielding the source of radiation with lead. The notion of half-value thickness introduced in Chapter 6 is very useful here. One half-thickness of absorber will reduce the exposure by one half, two half-thicknesses will reduce the exposure by an additional one fourth, *etc.* The half-value thicknesses of lead for a number of isotopes used in nuclear medicine are given in Table 9-2. An important number to remember is that 10 half-thicknesses will reduce the radiation exposure by a factor of 1,000. Thus, 2.5 mm. of lead will absorb 99.9% of the 140 keV gamma rays of ^{99m}Tc. This dose reduction is significant and important. It has been shown that a plastic disposable syringe containing 10 mCi of ^{99m}Tc delivers a radiation exposure of about 0.150 rad per minute at the surface of the syringe. The use of syringe shields should be mandatory in all nuclear medicine clinics, since these simple devices can reduce the exposure significantly.

Also listed in Table 9-2 are the dose factors for the radionuclides. The dose factor is the radiation exposure in milliroentgens per hour produced by a point source of one millicurie of the radionuclide at one meter (3.27 feet) from the source. This provides an indication of the radiation expo-

TABLE 9-2. — HALF-VALUE THICKNESSES OF LEAD FOR VARIOUS RADIONUCLIDES
USED IN NUCLEAR MEDICINE

RADIONUCLIDE	PRINCIPAL GAMMA-RAY ENERGY keV	DOSE FACTOR*	APPROXIMATE HALF-THICKNESS mm. of lead
99mTc	140	0.07	0.25
75Se	265	0.18	3.0
131I	364	0.22	6.0
113mIn	393	0.34	2.7
51Cr	320	0.15	1.8
198Au	412	0.23	2.8

*Dose Factor = milliroentgens per hour exposure from a point source of one millicurie at a distance of one meter (MR./MCi – hour).

sure to personnel at the 1-meter distance. Note that for a distance of 0.5 meter, the exposure increases by a factor of 4.0, and at 0.25 meter, exposure is increased by 16; this is the inverse-square law in action.

The radiation exposure from a distributed source, such as a patient containing radioactive material, is much more difficult to estimate accurately, but the dose rate factors of Table 9-2 can be applied to distributed sources at distances greater than about 1 meter. At closer distances, the actual distribution of the radioactive material in the patient can produce serious errors in the estimate.

The major problem in personnel protection, however, is not exposure from external sources, since most institutions provide adequate shielding for stocks of radioactive materials, but the hazards from internally deposited radionuclides. The nuclear medicine technician is continuously exposed to sizable quantities of radionuclides, and the possibilities for accidental ingestion are numerous. The most effective methods for preventing the internal deposition of radionuclides are extreme caution in handling vials, syringes and other containers to prevent personal contamination, and rigid rules prohibiting eating, drinking, and smoking in areas where radioisotopes are handled in any way. Personal cleanliness is also necessary to prevent radioactive contamination from being transferred from hands to food or drink. Most radionuclides used in radiopharmaceuticals for nuclear medicine are freely soluble in water, and simply washing the hands before eating will take care of most contamination hazards.

Waste Disposal and Decontamination

The safe disposal of radioactive waste materials is one of the most troublesome aspects of the nuclear age. Fortunately for nuclear medicine, most of the radionuclides used are relatively short-lived and their physical decay to stable nuclei essentially takes care of the problem. Most institutions are served by a commercial radioactive waste-disposal service, which often provides containers for all types of radioactive waste materials. These containers should be placed in the areas where waste material is generated (the preparation laboratory), and should be clearly marked. Avoid placing "cold" trash in the "hot" containers, since most disposal services charge by the pound or by volume.

The United States Atomic Energy Commission limits the amounts of radioactive materials which can be placed in sanitary sewer lines. However, there is no restriction at all on radioactive materials that have been used in humans in the diagnosis of diseases. Thus, blood samples from blood volume tests, urine samples from Schilling tests, and other biologic material may be disposed in the sanitary sewer system. For all other radioactive wastes, the concentrations of radionuclides which may be disposed of in sanitary sewer systems are listed in Handbook 69 of the National Committee on Radiation Protection, National Bureau of Standards. This handbook should be consulted regarding the limits on radioactive waste disposal, for it contains a wealth of information regarding maximum permissible body burdens of radionuclides as well as disposal procedures and limits.

Almost every laboratory has experienced a spill of radioactive materials resulting from a broken vial, sloppy handling of radioactive materials, or a patient who vomits after receiving an injection or oral dose of a radiopharmaceutical. Most spills can be cleaned up rather easily with soap, water, and plenty of absorbent material, provided the decontamination worker takes pains not to contaminate himself by wearing proper protective clothing, including rubber or plastic gloves. The greatest hazards arise from volatile materials, which quickly spread everywhere throughout the area. Although few radiopharmaceuticals are themselves volatile, there may be a hazard if the radioactive material becomes dry and then becomes airborne. The following general rules of procedure should be followed in the case of a spill of radioactive material:

1. Close off area to prevent contamination to or by unsuspecting persons.
2. Shut off ventilators and air conditioners.
3. Call the Radiation Protection Officer and tell him the extent and nature of the spill.
4. If unfamiliar with decontamination procedures, or if you don't know or are not sure of the type of radioactive material and/or the amount of material spilled, wait for the Radiation Safety Officer.
5. Proceed with decontamination by using protective clothing (rubber

150   *Nuclear Medicine for Technicians*

gloves, coveralls, shoe covers). Do not begin decontamination if airborne radioactivity is a possibility. Leave the area and seal doors with masking tape. Make certain there is no airflow into or out of the area.

6. Contain radioactive solutions to as small an area as possible. Use blotting paper, paper towel, or any absorbent material.
7. Keep area wet and covered with absorbent material. Blot up radioactive material, repeating until area is cold to survey or wipe tests. Dispose of all wastes in radioactive waste containers.

SUGGESTED READING

Blahd, W. H. (ed.): *Nuclear Medicine* (2d ed.; New York: McGraw-Hill Book Company, Inc., 1971), Chap. 1.
Johns, H. E.: *The Physics of Radiology* (2d ed.; Springfield, Ill.: Charles C Thomas, Publisher, 1964), Chaps. 9, 13, 17, 18.
National Committee on Radiation Protection: *Maximum Permissible Body Burdens and Maximum Permissible Concentrations of Radionuclides in Air and Water for Occupational Exposure* (National Bureau of Standards, Handbook 69). Quimby, E. H., Feitelberg, S., and Gross, W.: *Radioactive Nuclides in Medicine and Biology: Basic Physics and Instrumentation* (3d ed.; Philadelphia: Lea and Febiger, 1970), Chaps. 8-12.
Selman, J.: *The Fundamentals of X-Ray and Radium Physics* (4th ed.; Springfield, Ill.: Charles C Thomas, Publisher, 1965), Chap. 12.
Snell, A. H. (ed.): *Nuclear Instruments and Their Uses.* Vol. 1 (New York: John Wiley and Sons, Inc., 1962), Chaps. 6, 7.

STUDY QUESTIONS

1. Define the roentgen and the rad, and explain the difference between these units.
2. What is RBE and why is it necessary?
3. What are the sources of natural and artificial background radiation?
4. Discuss the differences in natural background exposure which depend on one's location on the earth.
5. What is the principal source of artificial background radiation?
6. What are the two biologic effects of ionizing radiation? Which do you believe to be more important in setting maximum permissible dose levels?
7. What is the difference between dominant and recessive mutations?
8. What is the doubling dose of ionizing radiation?
9. What is the annual MPD for workers exposed in the course of their jobs? For the general population?
10. Why may the hands, forearms, and feet be subjected to 15 times the annual radiation absorbed dose of the whole body?
11. What is the principal method presently used to monitor occupational exposure?
12. Discuss the similarities and differences between film badge and thermoluminescence dosimetry.
13. What are the three principles of minimizing exposure to ionizing radiation?

14. A source of ^{131}I containing 10 mCi of radioactivity was inadvertently placed in a lead shield 1.0 cm. thick, designed for ^{99m}Tc. Calculate the reduction in gamma-ray exposure produced by the shield for both isotopes.
15. List the procedures to be followed in the event of a spill of radioactive material.

Mathematics Review

THE PHYSICS OF NUCLEAR MEDICINE involves a fair amount of mathematic skill which is not difficult, but is easy to forget if not exercised regularly. Many of the numbers involved in the calculations of nuclear medicine are very large or very small, and mathematic shortcuts have been developed for handling these numbers with ease.

Exponential Notation

Almost all the numbers used in nuclear medicine have their origin in the metric system of measurement, which is basically the decimal system of measurement. The meter is the basic unit of length (1 meter = 39.3 inches), the liter, which is essentially 1,000 cubic centimeters, is the basic unit of volume (1 liter = 1.056 quart), and the gram is the basic unit of weight (1 gram = 0.035 ounce). In contrast with the familiar English system, which changes units as the measurement scale changes (ounces, pounds, tons for weight; inches, feet, yards and miles for length), the metric system simply adds a prefix to indicate multiplication by a constant factor. Thus, 1,000 grams is called one kilogram, and 1/1,000 of a gram is called a milligram. The presently used prefixes and their factors are given in Table A-1.

Exponential forms are used to write very large and very small numbers for mathematic operations. The exponential forms associated with

TABLE A-1.— METRIC PREFIXES AND THEIR MATHEMATIC EQUIVALENTS

PREFIX	ABBREVIATION	MULTIPLICATION FACTOR	EXPONENTIAL FORM
Pico-	p-	one trillionth	10^{-12}
Nano-	n-	one billionth	10^{-9}
Micro-	μ-	one millionth	10^{-6}
Milli-	m-	one thousandth	10^{-3}
Centi-	c-	one hundredth	10^{-2}
Kilo-	k-	one thousand	10^{3}
Mega-	M-	one million	10^{6}
Giga-	G-	one billion	10^{9}

the various metric prefixes are also given in Table A-1. One microcurie, in decimal form, would be written 0.000,001 curie, whereas the energy of the ^{99m}Tc gamma ray is written in decimal form as 140,000 ev. In exponential form, 1 μCi is written as 1×10^{-6} curie (read one times 10 to the minus six) and 140,000 is 140×10^3 ev (read 140 times 10 to the third). In this way, all quantities in physics can be expressed as a number between one and 1,000 multiplied by 10 raised to a power, saving the writing of a number of zeros. The speed of light, for example, is 30 billion centimeters per second, and is written 3×10^{10} cm./sec.

Addition and subtraction of exponential forms require that the exponents agree, as indicated in the following example. Add 1.575 mCi to 43 μCi:

$$1.575 \text{ mCi} = 1.575 \times 10^{-3} \text{ curie} = 1,575 \times 10^{-6} \text{ curie}$$
$$43 \ \mu\text{Ci} = \underline{\hspace{2cm} 43 \times 10^{-6} \text{ curie}}$$
$$\text{Sum} = 1,618 \times 10^{-6} \text{ curie.}$$

The answer, $1,618 \times 10^{-6}$ curie, may also be called 1.618 mCi or 1,618 μCi.

The basic rule for changing exponents is illustrated by the example above: moving the decimal point one place to the right requires the subtraction of 1 from the exponent; moving the decimal point one place to the left requires the addition of one to the exponent. This operation is illustrated below:

$$125.7 \times 10^{-6} = 12.57 \times 10^{-5} = 1.257 \times 10^{-4}$$

$$140.0 \times 10^3 \ = 14.00 \times 10^4 \ = 1.400 \times 10^5$$

$$3,700 \times 10^7 \ = 37.00 \times 10^9 \ = 3.700 \times 10^{10.}$$

Most mistakes which do occur in addition and subtraction of exponential numbers result from not making sure that the units are the same. Although it would appear at first glance that the addition of 1.75×10^{-6} meters to 5.43×10^{-6} cm. is simply 7.18×10^{-6}, the answer is incorrect; even though the exponents agree, the units are not the same. The problem is worked correctly below:

$$1.75 \times 10^{-6} \text{ meter} = 1.75 \times 10^{-6} \text{ meter} = 1.75 \times 10^{-6} \text{ meter}$$
$$+ \ 5.43 \times 10^{-6} \text{ cm.} \ = 5.43 \times 10^{-8} \text{ meter} = \underline{0.0543 \times 10^{-6} \text{ meter}}$$
$$\text{Sum} = 1.7643 \times 10^{-6} \text{ meter.}$$

Multiplication and division of exponential forms is also straightforward. First, perform the multiplication or division operation on the numerical part of the problem. Then, for multiplication, add the exponents algebraically; for division, subtract the exponent of the denominator from that of the numerator. Examples are provided below:

$(6.0 \times 10^5) \times (5.5 \times 10^4) = 33.0 \times 10^9 = 3.30 \times 10^{10}$

$(5.9 \times 10^4) \times (1.2 \times 10^{-3}) = 7.08 \times 10^1 = 70.8$

$(7.2 \times 10^5) \div (2.0 \times 10^7) = 3.60 \times 10^{-2}$

$(4.48 \times 10^{-7}) \div (8.0 \times 10^9) = 0.56 \times 10^{-16} = 5.6 \times 10^{-17}.$

Once again, many errors are made in attempting to divide one unit by a different unit of the same measure. Dividing meters by centimeters simply will not work.

Logarithms

Logarithms are another way of expressing very large and very small numbers. The logarithm (or log) of a number is the exponent or power to which the base must be raised to produce the number. Only two bases are used to any great extent, base 10 and base e (e, like pi, is a natural number which has a value of 2.71828). Four-place logs are tabulated in Appendix B.

First, let us consider only logs to base 10. The log of 2.00 is 0.3010. This means that $10^{0.3010}$ equals 2.00. The log of 3 is 0.4771; again, $10^{0.4771}$ equals 3.00. For numbers larger than 9, it is helpful to express the number in exponential form before attempting to find the log. For example, the log of 2,000 can be found by expressing 2000 as 2.000×10^3. The log of this number is $0.3010 + 3.00$, or 3.3010. Similarly, the log of 300 is the log of 3.00×10^2, or $0.4771 + 2.00$, or 2.4771. In these cases, $10^{3.3010}$ and $10^{2.4771}$ are equal to 2,000 and 300, respectively. A somewhat more difficult problem occurs for decimal numbers between 0 and 1, but may be solved by the same approach as used above for numbers larger than 9. For example, the log of 0.0020 is equal to the log of 2×10^{-3} or $0.3010 + (-3)$. This latter number can be expressed in a number of ways; usually the form is $7.3010 - 10$. Similarly, the log of 0.00003 is $5.4771 - 10$.

The examples provided above indicate two of the properties of logarithms: (1) The log of any number which can be written as 2.00×10^n will always include the log form 0.3010. This part of the logarithm is called the mantissa. (2) The other part of the log, which represents the exponential part of the number, is called the characteristic. Only mantissas are listed in tables of logarithms.

The base e (or 2.71828) is a useful base because many physical problems have solutions which include the value of e. For example, the equation expressing the amount of radioactive material remaining is

$$A = A_0 e^{-\lambda t}. \qquad \text{(A-1)}$$

Many tabulations of logs to base e exist, but since tables of logs to base 10 are much more common, a conversion factor is sometimes helpful:

$$\log_e = 2.303 \log_{10}. \tag{A-2}$$

Thus, $\log_e$ of 2.00 is $2.303 \times 0.3010 = 0.6932$.

Logarithms can be useful in solving a number of problems, if the mathematical rules for arithmetic operations are understood. These are given briefly in equation form below:

$$\log (A \times B) = \log A + \log B$$

$$\log (A \div B) = \log A - \log B \tag{A-3}$$

$$\log (A^B) = B \log A.$$

However, logs are not useful for addition and subtraction of numbers. Note that the log of (A + B) is *not* log A + log B. The addition (A + B) must be done before looking up the mantissa.

Logarithms can be usefully applied to simplify a number of exponential forms which are encountered in nuclear medicine calculations. Consider first equation A-1, which is $A = A_0 e^{-\lambda t}$. This equation can be rearranged (divide both sides by A_0) to give

$$\frac{A}{A_0} = e^{-\lambda t}. \tag{A-4}$$

Now, logs to base e are taken of both sides, giving

$$\log_e \left(\frac{A}{A_0}\right) = \log_e e^{-\lambda t}. \tag{A-5}$$

Using the rules of equation A-3, this can be reduced to

$$\log_e \left(\frac{A}{A_0}\right) = -\lambda t. \tag{A-6}$$

In words, equation A-6 reads that the $\log_e$ of the fraction of the activity remaining is equal to the negative product of the decay constant (λ) times the time.

Let us use equation A-6 to determine how much activity remains in a sample of ^{99m}Tc which contained 10.0 mCi 5 hours ago. The half life of ^{99m}Tc is 6.0 hours, so the decay constant (λ) is $-0.693/6.0 = 0.1155$ hour^{-1}. The product (λ) (t) is then $(0.511$ hour$^{-1} \times 5.0$ hour$) = 0.5775$, thus $\log_e \left(\frac{A}{A_0}\right)$ is -0.5775. Next we convert to base 10 by using equation A-3: $\log_{10} \frac{A}{A_0} = -0.5775/2.303 = -0.2505$. Since this is a negative mantissa and only positive values are listed in log tables, it must be converted to a positive mantissa and a negative characteristic. Here, -0.2505 is equal to $-1.0000 + 0.7495$, or $9.7495 - 10$. Looking up the mantissa 0.7495 in a log table, we find the number 5.617. Thus, $\dfrac{A}{A_0} = 5.617 \times 10^{-1}$, or 0.5617. This means that the fraction of ^{99m}Tc remaining after 5.0 hours is 0.5617, and the original 10.0-mCi sample now contains 5.617 mCi. These problems occur repeatedly in nuclear medicine, and the principle behind the calculations must be understood.

The original equation A-4 can be solved with a table of exponentials, such as included in Appendix C. To use equation A-4, all that is required is to multiply (λ) and (t), and look up the result in the table of exponents. Note that the table can be used to calculate the amount of activity present before the calibration time, by using $e^{+ \lambda t}$.

In the problem discussed above (i.e., what is the amount of ^{99m}Tc remaining in a sample 5 hours after it contained 10.0 mCi), the product (λ) (t) is -0.5775, or rounding off -0.58. Thus, the exponent to be looked up in the table is $e^{-0.58}$. Since this value is not listed in the table, we use the mathematic fact that $(e^x)(e^y) = e^{x+y}$, so that $e^{-0.58} = (e^{-0.5})(e^{-0.08})$. The tabular values are $e^{-0.5} = 0.607$ and $e^{-0.08} = 0.923$. Thus, $e^{-0.58} = (0.607)(0.923) = 0.560$, which is essentially the same answer as that obtained using logs.

For times before the calibration date, the positive exponentials are used. For example, to calculate the amount of ^{131}I in a sample 5 days before its calibration date, we again use equation A-4.

$$\frac{A}{A_0} = e^{-\lambda t}$$

Note that in this equation t is entered in the equation as a negative number ($t = 5$ days). For ^{131}I, $\lambda = \dfrac{0.693}{8.05d} = 0.0861$ day^{-1}. The product $-\lambda t = (-0.0861)(-5.0) = +0.4305$. Again rounding off, $-\lambda t = 0.43$, and from the table of exponentials, $e^{0.43} = e^{0.40} \times e^{0.03} = (1.492)(1.031) = 1.540$. Thus, if the ^{131}I contains 100 μCi on October 6, 5 days earlier, on October 1, the ^{131}I content was 154 μCi.

APPENDIX B
Four-Place Logarithms

N	0	1	2	3	4	5	6	7	8	9
10	0000	0043	0086	0128	0170	0212	0253	0294	0334	0374
11	0414	0453	0492	0531	0569	0607	0645	0682	0719	0755
12	0792	0828	0864	0899	0934	0969	1004	1038	1072	1106
13	1139	1173	1206	1239	1271	1303	1335	1367	1399	1430
14	1461	1492	1523	1553	1584	1614	1644	1673	1703	1732
15	1761	1790	1818	1847	1875	1903	1931	1959	1987	2014
16	2041	2068	2095	2122	2148	2175	2201	2227	2253	2279
17	2304	2330	2355	2380	2405	2430	2455	2480	2504	2529
18	2553	2577	2601	2625	2648	2672	2695	2718	2742	2765
19	2788	2810	2833	2856	2878	2900	2923	2945	2967	2989
20	3010	3032	3054	3075	3096	3118	3139	3160	3181	3201
21	3222	3243	3263	3284	3304	3324	3345	3365	3385	3404
22	3424	3444	3464	3483	3502	3522	3541	3560	3579	3598
23	3617	3636	3655	3674	3692	3711	3729	3747	3766	3784
24	3802	3820	3838	3856	3874	3892	3909	3927	3945	3962
25	3979	3997	4014	4031	4048	4065	4082	4099	4116	4133
26	4150	4166	4183	4200	4216	4232	4249	4265	4281	4298
27	4314	4330	4346	4362	4378	4393	4409	4425	4440	4456
28	4472	4487	4502	4518	4533	4548	4564	4579	4594	4609
29	4624	4639	4654	4669	4683	4698	4713	4728	4742	4757
30	4771	4786	4800	4814	4829	4843	4857	4871	4886	4900
31	4914	4928	4942	4955	4969	4983	4997	5011	5024	5038
32	5051	5065	5079	5092	5105	5119	5132	5145	5159	5172
33	5185	5198	5211	5224	5237	5250	5263	5276	5289	5302
34	5315	5328	5340	5353	5366	5378	5391	5403	5416	5428
35	5441	5453	5465	5478	5490	5502	5514	5527	5539	5551
36	5563	5575	5587	5599	5611	5623	5635	5647	5658	5670
37	5682	5694	5705	5717	5729	5740	5752	5763	5775	5786
38	5798	5809	5821	5832	5843	5855	5866	5877	5888	5899
39	5911	5922	5933	5944	5955	5966	5977	5988	5999	6010
40	6021	6031	6042	6053	6064	6075	6085	6096	6107	6117
41	6128	6138	6149	6160	6170	6180	6191	6201	6212	6222
42	6232	6243	6253	6263	6274	6284	6294	6304	6314	6325
43	6335	6345	6355	6365	6375	6385	6395	6405	6415	6425
44	6435	6444	6454	6464	6474	6484	6493	6503	6513	6522
45	6532	6542	6551	6561	6571	6580	6590	6599	6609	6618
46	6628	6637	6646	6656	6665	6675	6684	6693	6702	6712
47	6721	6730	6739	6749	6758	6767	6776	6785	6794	6803
48	6812	6821	6830	6839	6848	6857	6866	6875	6884	6893
49	6902	6911	6920	6928	6937	6946	6955	6964	6972	6981
50	6990	6998	7007	7016	7024	7033	7042	7050	7059	7067
51	7076	7084	7093	7101	7110	7118	7126	7135	7143	7152
52	7160	7168	7177	7185	7193	7202	7210	7218	7226	7235
53	7243	7251	7259	7267	7275	7284	7292	7300	7308	7316
54	7324	7332	7340	7348	7356	7364	7372	7380	7388	7396
55	7404	7412	7419	7427	7435	7443	7451	7459	7466	7474

N	0	1	2	3	4	5	6	7	8	9
56	7482	7490	7497	7505	7513	7520	7528	7536	7543	7551
57	7559	7566	7574	7582	7589	7597	7604	7612	7619	7627
58	7634	7642	7649	7657	7664	7672	7679	7686	7694	7701
59	7709	7716	7723	7731	7738	7745	7752	7760	7767	7774
60	7782	7789	7796	7803	7810	7818	7825	7832	7839	7846
61	7853	7860	7868	7875	7882	7889	7896	7903	7910	7917
62	7924	7931	7938	7945	7952	7959	7966	7973	7980	7987
63	7993	8000	8007	8014	8021	8028	8035	8041	8048	8055
64	8062	8069	8075	8082	8089	8096	8102	8109	8116	8122
65	8129	8136	8142	8149	8156	8162	8169	8176	8182	8189
66	8195	8202	8209	8215	8222	8228	8235	8241	8248	8254
67	8261	8267	8274	8280	8287	8293	8299	8306	8312	8319
68	8325	8331	8338	8344	8351	8357	8363	8370	8376	8382
69	8388	8395	8401	8407	8414	8420	8426	8432	8439	8445
70	8451	8457	8463	8470	8476	8482	8488	8494	8500	8506
71	8513	8519	8525	8531	8537	8543	8549	8555	8561	8567
72	8573	8579	8585	8591	8597	8603	8609	8615	8621	8627
73	8633	8639	8645	8651	8657	8663	8669	8675	8681	8686
74	8692	9698	8704	8710	8716	8722	8727	8733	8739	8745
75	8751	8756	8762	8768	8774	8779	8785	8791	8797	8802
76	8808	8814	8820	8825	8831	8837	8842	8848	8854	8859
77	8865	8871	8876	8882	8887	8893	8899	8904	8910	8915
78	8921	8927	8932	8938	8943	8949	8954	8960	8965	8971
79	8976	8982	8987	8993	8998	9004	9009	9015	9020	9025
80	9031	9036	9042	9047	9053	9058	9063	9069	9074	9079
81	9085	9090	9096	9101	9106	9112	9117	9122	9128	9133
82	9138	9143	9149	9154	9159	9165	9170	9175	9180	9186
83	9191	9196	9201	9206	9212	9217	9222	9227	9232	9238
84	9243	9248	9253	9258	9263	9269	9274	9279	9284	9289
85	9294	9299	9304	9309	9315	9320	9325	9330	9335	9340
86	9345	9350	9355	9360	9365	9370	9375	9380	9385	9390
87	9395	9400	9405	9410	9415	9420	9425	9430	9435	9440
88	9445	9450	9455	9460	9465	9469	9474	9479	9484	9489
89	9494	9499	9504	9509	9513	9518	9523	9528	9533	9538
90	9542	9547	9552	9557	9562	9566	9571	9576	9581	9586
91	9590	9595	9600	9605	9609	9614	9619	9624	9628	9633
92	9638	9643	9647	9652	9657	9661	9666	9671	9675	9680
93	9685	9689	9694	9699	9703	9708	9713	9717	9722	9727
94	9731	9736	9741	9745	9750	9754	9759	9763	9768	9773
95	9777	9782	9786	9791	9795	9800	9805	9809	9814	9818
96	9823	9827	9832	9836	9841	9845	9850	9854	9859	9863
97	9868	9872	9877	9881	9886	9890	9894	9899	9903	9908
98	9912	9917	9921	9926	9930	9934	9939	9943	9948	9952
99	9956	9961	9965	9969	9974	9978	9983	9987	9991	9996

APPENDIX C

Exponentials

x	e^{-x}	e^{+x}	x	e^{-x}	e^{+x}
0.01	.990	1.010	1.0	0.368	2.718
0.02	.980	1.020	2.0	0.135	7.38
0.03	.970	1.031	3.0	0.0498	20.0
0.04	.961	1.041	4.0	0.0183	54.5
0.05	.951	1.052	5.0	0.0067	147.8
0.06	.942	1.062	6.0	0.0025	400.0
0.07	.932	1.073	7.0	0.0009	1090.
0.08	.923	1.083	8.0	0.0003	2970.
0.09	.914	1.094	9.0	0.0001	8050.
0.10	0.905	1.105			
0.20	0.819	1.222			
0.30	0.741	1.350			
0.40	0.670	1.492			
0.50	0.607	1.670			
0.60	0.549	1.822			
0.70	0.497	2.015			
0.80	0.449	2.23			
0.90	0.407	2.46			

Physical Characteristics of Radionuclides Used in Nuclear Medicine

Radionuclide	Half-Life ($t_{1/2}$)	Decay Constant (λ)	Principal Gamma Rays
^{3}H	12.26 years	0.0565 year^{-1}	no gammas; $E^{\beta}_{max} = 17.5$ keV
^{14}C	5,600 years	0.000124 year^{-1}	no gammas; $E^{\beta}_{max} = 156$ keV
^{18}F	1.87 hours	0.370 hour^{-1}	511 keV (annihilation radiation)
^{32}P	14.3 days	0.0484 day^{-1}	no gammas; $E^{\beta}_{max} = 1.71$ MeV
^{42}K	12.49 hours	0.0556 hour^{-1}	1.53 MeV
^{47}Ca	4.9 days	0.141 day^{-1}	1.31 MeV
^{51}Cr	27.8 days	0.0249 day^{-1}	320 keV
^{59}Fe	45.1 days	0.0154 day^{-1}	1.10, 1.29 MeV
^{57}Co	270 days	0.00256 day^{-1}	122 keV
^{60}Co	5.3 years	0.131 year^{-1}	1.17, 1.33 MeV
^{65}Zn	245 days	0.00283 day^{-1}	1.114 MeV
^{67}Ga	78 hours	0.00889 hour^{-1}	182,296 keV
^{75}Se	127 days	0.00546 day^{-1}	265, 136, 280 keV
^{85}Kr	10.6 years	0.0654 year^{-1}	520 keV
^{86}Rb	18.6 days	0.0373 day^{-1}	1.08 MeV
^{85}Sr	65.0 days	0.0107 day^{-1}	513 keV
^{87}Y	80 hours	0.00867 hour^{-1}	parent of ^{87m}Sr
^{87m}Sr	2.80 hours	0.247 hour^{-1}	388 keV
^{99}Mo	67.0 hours	0.01033 hour^{-1}	parent of ^{99m}Tc
^{99m}Tc	6.0 hours	0.1155 hour^{-1}	140 keV
^{113}Sn	115 days	0.00602 day	parent of ^{113m}In
^{113m}In	1.75 hours	0.396 hour^{-1}	393 keV
^{123}I	13.0 hours	0.0532 hour^{-1}	159 keV
^{125}I	60.0 days	0.0115 day^{-1}	28 keV (Te K-characteristic x-rays)
^{131}I	8.05 days	0.0861 day^{-1}	364 keV
^{133}Xe	5.27 days	0.1314 day^{-1}	81 keV
^{131}Ba	11.6 days	0.0597 day^{-1}	122, 214, 372 keV
^{133m}Ba	38.8 hours	0.01787 hour^{-1}	276 keV
^{144}Ce	290 days	0.00239 day^{-1}	134, 81 keV
^{198}Au	2.70 days	0.256 day^{-1}	412 keV

Index